CORPVS MEDICORVM GRAECORVM

EDIDIT

ACADEMIA BEROLINENSIS ET BRANDENBVRGENSIS
CVM ACADEMIIS HAVNIENSI ATQVE LIPSIENSI

I 4,1

HIPPOCRATIS

DE CAPITIS VVLNERIBVS

EDIDIT, IN LINGVAM ANGLICAM VERTIT,
COMMENTATVS EST

MAURY HANSON

IN AEDIBVS ACADEMIAE SCIENTIARVM

HIPPOCRATES

ON HEAD WOUNDS

EDITION, TRANSLATION AND COMMENTARY
BY
MAURY HANSON

AKADEMIE VERLAG

Dieser Band wurde durch die Bund-Länder-Kommission für Bildungsplanung
und Forschungsförderung im Akademienprogramm mit Mitteln des Bundes (Bundesministerium
für Bildung, Wissenschaft, Forschung und Technologie) und des Landes Berlin
(Senatsverwaltung für Wissenschaft, Forschung und Kultur) gefördert.

Die Deutsche Bibliothek - CIP-Einheitsaufnahme

Hippocrates:
[De capitis vulneribus]
Hippocratis De capitis vulneribus / ed., in linguam Anglicam vertit,
commentatus est Maury Hanson. - Berlin : Akad. Verl., 1999
(Corpus medicorum Graecorum ; 1,4,1)
ISBN 3-05-003339-8

ISSN 0070-0347

Der Akademie Verlag ist ein Unternehmen der R. Oldenbourg-Gruppe.

Das eingesetzte Papier ist alterungsbeständig nach DIN/ISO 9706.

Druck und Bindung: Druckhaus „Thomas Müntzer“, Bad Langensalza

Printed in the Federal Republic of Germany

TO MY PARENTS

PREFACE

For fellowship support of the initial phases of this project I am indebted to the Hannah Institute for the History of Medicine.

An especial debt of gratitude is owed to Richard Durling, who suggested the project to me. I would also like to thank Paul Potter, whose personal library was a great boon, and Beate Gundert for their help and hospitality during my stay in Canada. Libraries have, of course, provided the place and the material for much of my work, and I would like to express my gratitude in particular to Father Leonard E. Boyle, O.P., Prefect of the Vatican Library, Dr. Anna Lenzuni, Director of the Laurentian Library, Professor Donald Russell and Mr. Nigel Wilson from whose friendly counsel I benefitted during my work at the Bodleian Library, Mrs. Dorothy Hanks and Miss Margaret Kaiser and their staff of the History of Medicine Division of the National Library of Medicine, and to the staff of the Weldon Library of the University of Western Ontario. The knowledge and willing advice of all these people improved my work and also made it easier and more enjoyable.

In the final stages of this work the advice and guidance of the editorial staff of the Corpus Medicorum Graecorum, especially Jutta Kollesch and Diethard Nickel, have been invaluable, improving both shape and substance.

My thanks go also to the Berlin-Brandenburgische Akademie der Wissenschaften for the decision to include my edition in the series of the Corpus Medicorum Graecorum.

Finally, I owe especial thanks to my friends, Rosemary Howard and Richard Lykes, for their help and support, which has always been generously given, especially during those periods when the project kept me away from home.

Woodbourne, Madison County, Virginia Maury Hanson
March 1998

TABLE OF CONTENTS

BIBLIOGRAPHY[1]

B. Alexanderson, Die hippokratische Schrift Prognostikon. Überlieferung und Text, Göteborg, 1963 (Studia Graeca et Latina Gothoburgensia XVII)

A. P. Bagliani, La provenienza 'angioina' dei codici greci della biblioteca di Bonifacio VIII, Italia Medioevale e Umanistica 26, 1983, pp. 27–69

J. Bertier, Mnésithée et Dieuchès, Leiden, 1972 (Philosophia antiqua 20)

P. Canart, Le livre grec en Italie Méridionale sous les règnes Normand et Souabe: aspects matériels et sociaux, Scrittura e Civiltà 2, 1978, pp. 103–162

A. Cornelii Celsi quae supersunt, ed. F. Marx, CML I, Leipzig and Berlin, 1915

CMG = Corpus Medicorum Graecorum

CML = Corpus Medicorum Latinorum

A. Cocchi, Veterum medicorum chirurgica quaedam antehac desiderata, Florence, 1754

J. D. Denniston, The Greek particles, 2nd ed., Oxford, 1954 (repr. 1978)

R. Devreesse, Le fond grec de la Bibliothèque Vaticane des origines à Paul V, Studi e Testi 244, Rome, 1965

H. Diller see Hippocratis De aere aquis locis

F. Ehrle, Historia Bibliothecae Romanorum Pontificum tum Bonifatianae tum Avenionensis, I, Rome, 1890

Erotiani Vocum Hippocraticarum conlectio, ed. J. Klein, Leipzig, 1865

Erotiani Vocum Hippocraticarum collectio cum fragmentis, ed. E. Nachmanson, Uppsala, 1918

Claudii Galeni Opera omnia, ed. C. G. Kühn, 20 vols., Leipzig, 1821–1833 (= K.)

Claudii Galeni Pergameni Scripta minora, vol. II, ed. I. Müller, Leipzig, 1891

Galeni De usu partium libri XVII, ed. G. Helmreich, 2 vols., Leipzig, 1907/1909

Galeni In Hippocratis De victu acutorum comm. IV, ed. G. Helmreich, in: CMG V 9,1, Leipzig and Berlin, 1914

Galeni In Hippocratis Epidemiarum libr. III comm. III, ed. E. Wenkebach, CMG V 10,2,1, Leipzig and Berlin, 1936

–, In Hippocratis Epidemiarum libr. VI comm. I–VI, ed. E. Wenkebach; comm. VI–VIII, transl. F. Pfaff, CMG V 10,2,2, 2nd ed., Berlin, 1956

E. Gamillscheg and D. Harlfinger, Repertorium der griechischen Kopisten 800–1600, I. Teil: Handschriften aus Bibliotheken Großbritanniens, A: Verzeichnis der Kopisten, Vienna, 1981; II. Teil: Handschriften aus Bibliotheken Frankreichs, A: Verzeichnis der Kopisten, Vienna, 1989

Œuvres complètes d'Hippocrate, ed. and transl. E. Littré, 10 vols., Paris, 1839–1861 (= L.)

Hippocratis Opera quae feruntur omnia, ed. H. Kühlewein, 2 vols., Leipzig, 1894/1902 (= Kw.)

Hippocratis De prisca medicina, De liquidorum usu, ed. J. L. Heiberg, in: CMG I 1, Leipzig and Berlin, 1927

Hippocratis De aere aquis locis, ed. and transl. H. Diller, CMG I 1,2, Berlin, 1970

1 Works cited once are described in full in the appropriate place.

Hippocratis De natura hominis, ed., transl., and comm. J. Jouanna, CMG I 1,3, Berlin, 1975

Hippocrates with an English translation, vol. III, ed. E. T. Withington, London and Cambridge, Mass., 1928 (Loeb Classical Library)

Hippokrates, Über Entstehung und Aufbau des menschlichen Körpers (Περὶ σαρκῶν), ed., transl., and comm. K. Deichgräber, Leipzig and Berlin, 1935

Hippocratis De morbis I see Wittern

Ḥunain ibn Isḥāq, Über die syrischen und arabischen Galen-Übersetzungen, ed. and transl. G. Bergsträßer, Leipzig, 1925 (Abh. f. d. Kunde d. Morgenlandes 17,2)

J. Ilberg, Zur Überlieferung des Hippokratischen Corpus, Rheinisches Museum 42, 1887, pp. 436–461

–, Prolegomena I: De codicibus manu scriptis, in: Hippocratis Opera, ed. H. Kühlewein, I, pp. V–XXVIII

Index Hippocraticus see J.-H. Kühn and U. Fleischer

J. Irigoin, L'Italie méridionale et la tradition des textes antiques, Jahrbuch der Österreichischen Byzantinistik 18, 1969, pp. 37–55

–, Tradition manuscrite et histoire du texte: quelques problèmes relatifs à la Collection hippocratique, Revue d'Histoire des Textes 3, 1973, pp. 1–13 (also in: La Collection hippocratique et son rôle dans l'histoire de la médecine. Colloque de Strasbourg [23–27 octobre 1972], ed. L. Bourgey and J. Jouanna, Leiden, 1975 [Université des Sciences Humaines de Strasbourg, Travaux du Centre de Recherche sur le Proche-Orient et la Grèce antiques 2], pp. 3–18)

J. Jouanna see Hippocratis De natura hominis

F. Kudlien, Die handschriftliche Überlieferung des Galenkommentars zu Hippokrates De articulis, Berlin, 1960 (Deutsche Akademie d. Wiss. zu Berlin, Schriften d. Sektion f. Altertumswiss. 27)

H. Kühlewein see Hippocratis Opera

J.-H. Kühn and U. Fleischer, Index Hippocraticus. Cui elaborando interfuerunt sodales Thesauri Linguae Graecae Hamburgensis, curas postremas adhibuerunt K. Alpers, A. Anastassiou, D. Irmer, V. Schmidt, fasc. I–IV, Göttingen, 1986–1989

C. Lienau, Hippocratis De superfetatione, ed., transl., and comm., CMG I 2,2, Berlin, 1973

LSJ = H. G. Liddell, R. Scott, H. S. Jones, A Greek-English Lexicon, 9th ed., Oxford, 1940

J. Mercati and P. Franchi de' Cavalieri, Codices Vaticani Graeci, I, Rome, 1923

B. Mondrain, Un manuscrit d'Hippocrate: Le Monacensis graecus 71 et son histoire aux XVe et XVIe siècles, Revue d'Histoire des Textes 18, 1988, pp. 201–214

H. Omont, Catalogues des manuscrits grecs de Fontainebleau sous François Ier et Henri II, Paris, 1889

Oribasii Collectionum medicarum reliquiae, ed. J. Raeder, CMG VI 2,1, Leipzig and Berlin, 1931

Pauli Aeginetae Libri V–VII, ed. J. L. Heiberg, CMG IX 2, Leipzig and Berlin, 1924

J. E. Petrequin, Chirurgie d'Hippocrate, vol. I, Paris, 1877

A. Rivier, Recherches sur la tradition manuscrite du traité hippocratique «De morbo sacro», Berne, 1962 (Travaux publiés sous les auspices de la Société Suisse des Sciences Morales 3)

Œuvres de Rufus d'Ephèse, ed. and transl. Ch. Daremberg and Ch. E. Ruelle, Paris, 1879

H. Schöne, Apollonius von Kitium, Illustrierter Kommentar zu der hippokratischen Schrift Περὶ ἄρθρων, ed., Leipzig, 1896

K. Schubring, in: Hippokrates, Über Entstehung und Aufbau des menschlichen Körpers

Sorani De signis fracturarum, ed. J. Ilberg, in: CMG IV, Leipzig and Berlin, 1927

H. Stevenson, Codices manuscripti Palatini Graeci Bibliothecae Vaticanae, Rome, 1885

M. Wellmann, Die Fragmente der sikelischen Ärzte Akron, Philistion und des Diokles von Karystos, Berlin, 1901 (Fragmentsammlung der griechischen Ärzte I)

E. T. Withington see Hippocrates with an English translation

R. Wittern, Die hippokratische Schrift De morbis I. Ausgabe, Übersetzung und Erläuterungen, Hildesheim and New York, 1974

INTRODUCTION

A. The sources for the text

I. Greek manuscripts

Nine Greek manuscripts contain the text of De capitis vulneribus[1]:

Laurentianus Gr. 74,7	s. X	B
Vaticanus Gr. 276	s. XII	V
Palatinus Gr. 192	s. XV	P
Monacensis Gr. 71	s. XV	Mo
Parisinus Gr. 2146	s. XVI	C
Holkhamensis Gr. 92	s. XVI	Ho
Parisinus Gr. 2248	s. XVI	N
Parisinus Gr. 2247	s. XVI	M
Parisinus Gr. 2255	s. XVI	E

a) Laurentianus Gr. 74,7

Laurentianus Gr. 74,7 (= B)[2] is a vellum codex (370 x 270 mm) containing on 405 folios a collection of surgical writings extending from classical antiquity to the 7th c. Its compilation is attributed to Nicetas, a physician of Constantinople, who is credited, in the verses which precede the texts, with restoring interest in the ancient physicians. According to an inscription at the end of the volume (see below, p. 15) it belonged at one point to the Hospital **B**

1 See H. Diels, Die Handschriften der antiken Ärzte, I. Teil: Hippokrates und Galenos, Abh. d. Königl. Preuß. Akademie d. Wiss. 1905, phil.-hist. Kl. 3, Berlin, 1905, p. 10. In addition, a single sentence from De cap. vuln. (p. 90,5–6) is quoted in the 16th c. manuscript Vaticanus Gr. 2246 which consists of the notes of George Balsamon (see S. Lilla, Codices Vaticani Graeci [codices 2162–2254], Rome, 1985, pp. 398–399). It contains on fol. 4^{r} the following entry: ἱπποκράτου ἐν τῷ περὶ τῶν ἐν κεφαλῇ τρωμάτων· τὸ δὲ φάρμακον χρὴ διδόναι πρὸς τὴν δύναμιν τοῦ ἀνθρώπου ὁρῶν, ὡς ἂν ἰσχύος ἔχῃ. – P. Kibre, Hippocrates Latinus. Repertorium of Hippocratic writings in the Latin Middle Ages, revised edition, New York, 1985, p. 234, lists two Latin manuscripts as containing fragments of anonymous translations of De cap. vuln.: Monacensis Lat. 161, s. XII/XIII, fol. 39^{r}–46^{v}, and Monacensis Lat. 614, s. XIII, fol. 2^{r}–9^{r}. However, neither manuscript provides a translation of even a part of this Hippocratic text, nor does either show any definite influence of it. – The treatise was not translated into Syriac or Arabic. Ḥunayn ibn Isḥāq points out in his missive that no manuscript of the Greek text was available to him; see Ḥunain, no. 94; cf. below, p. 37 n. 1.

2 For a detailed description of this manuscript see Schöne, pp. V–XX; cf. A. M. Bandini, Catalogus Manuscriptorum Graecorum Bibliothecae Laurentianae, III, Florence, 1770 (repr. Leipzig, 1961), cols. 53–93.

of the 40 Martyrs in Constantinople.[1] The next record of the manuscript is found in two documents of the 15th c.: a list preserved in a manuscript of the former Royal Library of Hanover, "Auctores graeci: quos impensis Laurentii Medicis Lascaris ex peloponneso in Italiam nuper advexit"[2] and a contract, preserved in the Medicean Archives in Florence, drawn between Lascaris and Niccolò di Giacomo of Siena on 2 April 1492 in Candia, Crete.[3] The list, which contains orthographical and grammatical errors, provides a clear description of B, "Liber magnus aliquis in quo depicta sunt omnia genera ligaminum et Juncturarum. Correctiones cum necessariis instrumentis", with a list of its authors; the contract specifies, among those books apparently supplied in Crete, "Ipocratis et aliorum de ligaminibus et dislocacionibus". Whatever its exact route from Constantinople may have been, B appears to have been acquired by Lascaris while travelling expressly to buy books for Lorenzo the Magnificent and to have been brought to Florence by him in 1492. The expulsion of the Medici from Florence in 1494 and, a few years later, the rampage of Savonarola caused several moves within Florence for the Medici library. Then in 1508 it was brought to Rome on the order of Cardinal Giovanni de' Medici, later Pope Leo X. After the death of Leo X in 1521 the collection came under the protection of Cardinal Giulio de' Medici who became Pope Clement VII in 1523. On his order the books were returned to Florence in 1527 and a permanent home provided for them.[4] The Laurentian Library was dedicated by Clement VII in 1532. B, however, was again brought to Rome in 1534 on the order of Clement VII for study by Lascaris.[5] After Clement's death B remained in Rome in the library of Cardinal Niccolò Ridolfi, a relative of the Medici. Here it was used around 1540 by Guido Guidi in making his Latin translations of some of the treatises.[6] The route by which B was returned to Florence and the date of its return are not known.

B has two columns per page. The hand is a large, clear and beautiful minuscule, with neat, rounded letters, each about 3 mm in height. Accents and breathings in the hand of the scribe are few and very small. As a result of more recent studies B may now be dated with reasonable certainty to the 10th

1 A hospital of this name is said to have been founded by the emperor Isaac Angelus in Constantinople in 1190 (see Cocchi, p. 42). If B belonged to that hospital it would, of course, have had an earlier owner. However, the words for "40 Martyrs" are missing in the note at the back of the manuscript, and it is quite possible that B was owned by a different hospital.

2 See E. G. Vogel, Litterarische Ausbeute von Janus Lascaris' Reisen im Peloponnes um's Jahr 1490, Serapeum 2, 1854, pp. 154–160.

3 See E. Piccolomini, Due documenti relativi ad acquisti di codici greci, fatti da Giovanni Lascaris per conto di Lorenzo de' Medici, Rivista di Filologia e d'Istruzione Classica 2, 1874, pp. 401–423; id., Aggiunte e rettificazioni, Rivista di Filologia e d'Istruzione Classica 3, 1875, pp. 150–152.

4 See K. K. Müller, Neue Mittheilungen über Janos Laskaris und die Mediceische Bibliothek, Centralblatt für Bibliothekswesen 1, 1884, p. 349.

5 See Schöne, p. XVII.

6 See the note of Guido Guidi in Paris. Lat. 6866, fol. 264^{v}: Extat in bibliotheca Cardinalis Rodulphi ... graecus codex vetustissimus, in quo cum plures alii clarissimorum medicorum super chirurgia, tum libri tres de fasciis continentur. ...

century.[1] Large accents, breathings and marginal notes have been added in two later hands: B^2, light brown, irregular and quite careless in comparison to B^2 the main hand, and B^3, in a darker ink. Kühlewein dated these hands to 11th– B^3 12th and 14th c. respectively.[2]

Originally B contained six Hippocratic treatises: Κατ' ἰητρεῖον, Περὶ ἀγμῶν, Περὶ ἄρϑρων, Περὶ τῶν ἐν κεφαλῇ τρωμάτων, Μοχλικόν, and Περὶ ὀστέων φύσιος. However, a number of consecutive folios have been lost,[3] beginning in ch. 16 of De capitis vulneribus, whose last words in B are ἐν τῷ ὀ(στέῳ) (p. 84,25). These words occur in the last line of fol. 81^v. There is marked discoloration, which looks like liquid damage, at the top of the folio which now follows De capitis vulneribus, suggesting that the missing folios were discarded because of that damage. In addition to the last chapters of De capitis vulneribus, the two treatises which followed De capitis vulneribus, Mochlikon and De ossium natura, were also lost.[4] On fol. 407^v of the manuscript an inscription occurs, which is restored by the 18th c. editor, Cocchi, as follows: ⟨τὸ⟩ παρὸν ⟨βι⟩βλίον ὑπάρχει τοῦ ⟨ἰατρείου⟩ τοῦ νοσοκομείου τῶν ⟨μ' μαρτύρων·⟩ ἔχει δὲ φύλλα ⟨τετρα⟩κόσια εἴκοσι πέντε μηνὶ Μαίῳ ⟨ἰνδικτιῶ⟩νος ἕκτης.[5] In a later hand, possibly 14th c., above this inscription occurs the comment, Ἡ παροῦσα βίβλος ἔχει φύλλα υγ'. Therefore the loss of text occurred at the latest in the 14th c. before the manuscript was brought by Lascaris to Florence.[6] The remnant of the treatise De capitis vulneribus occurs on folios 75ra to 81vb.

B shows the following types of errors:

1. Omissions, for example

More extensive omissions, in part caused by adjacent wording (often, for

1 See Kudlien, pp. 11–12; K. Weitzmann, Die byzantinische Buchmalerei des 9. und 10. Jahrhunderts, Berlin, 1935, p. 33; cf. also N. G. Wilson, Aspects of the transmission of Galen, in: Le strade del testo, ed. G. Cavallo, Bari, 1987, pp. 51–52.

2 This dating is reported by Ilberg, Prolegomena, p. XV. However, some of the corrections may be later. Kudlien, pp. 15–17, points out that some textual corrections agree with Paris. Gr. 1849 and some with the sense of Vidius' translation and that these corrections may have been made by Vidius and by Lascaris or one of his students since Lascaris had both Paris. Gr. 1849 and B in his possession.

3 For a chart of the present order of folios and the extent of loss see Schöne, pp. VI–IX.

4 Irigoin, Tradition, pp. 3–4; 9–10 (= pp. 7; 12–13), pointed out that the first four of the six Hippocratic treatises of B are found also in V and in the same order both in the index and in the manuscript, while the two lost from B occur together only in the index at a later place, and the four that are common to both manuscripts are the four on which Galen prepared commentaries. Irigoin's thesis here is that the collections of Hippocratic works, i.e. their arrangement in codices, which we have today were products not of the Alexandrian period but of the 10th c. He conceded that the arrangement noted for these four treatises does not imply that B is the model for V. F. Pfaff, Die Überlieferung des Corpus Hippocraticum in der nachalexandrinischen Zeit, Wiener Studien 50, 1932, pp. 75–76, noting the lack in B of readings from the text of Artemidorus, concluded that B alone of the five early Hippocratic manuscripts is not based on the text of Artemidorus and is of a tradition independent from that of V.

5 See Cocchi, p. 42.

6 For the bad condition of the manuscript at this time see Schöne, p. XVII n. 16.

example, by homoioteleuton), were corrected in several instances by B² by means of marginal notes:

p. 66,1 ἐν^II – 2 ἀποθανεῖται om. B, in marg. add. B²
p. 72,1 καὶ – 2 ἐσφλασθέντα om. B
p. 78,9 ἢ – δεξάμενος om. B
p. 80,13 ἢν – 14 ἐπιλαμβάνει om. B
p. 82,4 ἢ – φλάσις^II om. B, in marg. add. B²
p. 82,11 καὶ – ἐτρώθη om. B, in marg. add. B²

Omissions of shorter segments of text or of single words are seen in these examples: p. 62,11 ἢ; p. 62,12 πρὸ; p. 68,26 τῇ τε ῥωγμῇ; p. 74,4 ἂν; p. 78,19 ἡ ἄλλη.

2. Additions, for example

p. 68,25 ante ἐγγενομένης add. ἂν B
p. 76,16 ante ἕδρη^I add. ἡ B
p. 76,19 ἡ bis scr. B
p. 80,27 post σίνασθαι add. τὴν σαρκα B
p. 82,6 post καὶ add. ου δη B
p. 84,8 ante περισφίγγηται add. ιωμενον B
p. 84,24 ante ἕλκεος add. ἐξ B

3. Transposition of words

p. 64,5 πολλὰ καὶ ὑγρά] ὑγρὰ και πολλὰ B
p. 64,16 ἐστι post χαλεπώτερα trsp. B
p. 74,10 μᾶλλον post χωρίου trsp. B
p. 74,11–12 βέλεα τιτρώσκει] τιτρωσκει βελεα B
p. 76,22 ὀστέα post περιέχοντα trsp. B

4. Wrong readings, for example

p. 62,3 σφίσιν] φησὶν B
p. 66,11 δὲ γίνονται] δ' ἐπιγίνονται B
p. 68,1 πόνων] ποιεων B
p. 68,13 ἐστι τὴν ἰδέην] ἐστιν· ἡ δὲ B
p. 70,10 βραχυτέρη] μηκροτερη B
p. 74,13 σκληρότατόν] επισκληροτατον B
p. 76,26 ῥαφὰς] σαρκας B
p. 80,3 ἑλκέων] ὀστεων B

Further errors concern: wrong inflectional endings (p. 62,21 ἀφήκουσα] ἀφηκουσαν; p. 66,4 ἐλάσσων ταύτῃ] ελασσω ταυτης; p. 66,21 τῇ ῥωγμῇ] τῆς ῥώγμης; p. 74,2 τρῶσαι] τρωσαν; p. 78,7 πολὺ] πολλω; p. 80,17 τὴν τομήν] της τομης), mistakes in degrees of comparison (p. 66,26 λεπταὶ] λεπτοταται; p. 74,10 μαλθακώτερον] μαλθακοτατον; p. 76,23 ἰσχυρότερά] ισχυροτατα), wrong word divisions (p. 74,9 δ' ἐξ ἰσοπέδου] δεξιω πεδου; p. 80,22 μάζῃ ἐκ λεπτῶν] μαζης κλεπτων (caused by error in the reading of uncial script, C for Є); p. 82,7 ὥρης, ἢν] ὡρησιν), synonym variants (p. 72,2 κέχρηται] δειται; p. 72,19 κακὸν] νοσημα), orthographic mistakes (for example, iotacism: p. 62,6 πεφυκυῖαι] πεφυκοιαι; p. 62,18 μηδετέρωϑι] μηδετερωϑη; p. 66,25 ἰδέαι] εἴδεαι; p. 70,16 τῇ^{II}] τοι; p. 70,17 εἴη] ηι; p. 72,24 ἐξελέγχειν] εξελεγχην; p. 76,1 κοπείσας] κοπησας; p. 80,2 τινὸς] τεινος; p. 84,16 ὑποπύους] ὑποποιους; confusion of αι and ε: p. 62,16 γραμμέων] γραμμαιων; p. 66,9 ἕδραι] ἀιδραι; p. 74,6 τιτρώσκονται] τιτρωσκοντε; p. 84,14 φλεγμαίνοι] φλεγμενοι; confusion of ο and ω: p. 66,1 ἄλλως] αλλος; p. 74,12 ἐμπεσὸν] ἐμπεσων; p. 76,3 ὡσαύτως] ὡσαυτος; p. 78,7 πολλὸν] πολλων).

Other peculiarities of B:

1. Iota adscript

Iota subscript does not appear, but iota adscript is frequent, e.g.: p. 72,23 λογωι; p. 72,24 εργωι; p. 74,5 βάλληι; p. 84,11 εωυτεηι.

2. ν ἐφελκυστικόν

There is rather frequent use of ν ἐφελκυστικόν, even before consonants, e.g.: p. 62,18 τησιν μακρησι γραμμησιν; p. 62,22 ἐστιν το οστεον; p. 68,15 τοισιν ὀφϑαλμοισιν καταφανὲς; p. 70,21 πεπονϑεν το κακον.

b) Vaticanus Gr. 276

Vaticanus Gr. 276 (= V) is a large (395 x 277 mm) vellum manuscript of V the 12th c., comprising II + 207 folios. It contains an index and 35 Hippocratic works.[1] The index, however, contains 62 works, differing from the manuscript not only in listing works not present, but also in failing to list two works, Περὶ διαίτης ὀξέων and Δόγμα Ἀϑηναίων, in listing Περὶ ἐπικυήσιος only once, and in placing some of the works in a different sequence.[2] Of the Hippocratic manuscripts which survive from the Middle Ages only Marcianus Gr. 269 matches V in its apparent attempt to provide a large selection of Hippocratic writings, i.e. to present the Hippocratic corpus rather than a section of it.

The earliest secure evidence for the provenance of V is found in the Vatican Library records where V is described as among manuscripts lent to Cardinal Bessarion from 1455 to 1458 and not returned on time.[3] V is again described in the inventories of Sixtus IV of 1475 and 1481.[4] The earlier history of V is less certain. In the 13th c. it may have been in the library of the Norman and then Hohenstaufen kings of Sicily. Following the defeat of Manfred at the battle of Benevento in 1266, it is possible that V, along with other manuscripts from the Norman collection, was given to pope Clement IV, by Charles of Anjou. The evidence for this provenance, far from conclusive, is threefold. First, the abbreviation "And." appears twice on the first folio of

1 This count includes two entries for one treatise, Περὶ ἐπικυήσιος, which appears twice. Only entire works are counted, e.g. Ἐπιδημίαι is counted as one, not seven.

2 For the description of this manuscript see Ilberg, Überlieferung, pp. 444–448; id., Prolegomena, pp. XV–XVIII; Lienau, pp. 13–18; Mercati and Franchi de' Cavalieri, pp. 362–365.

3 See Devreesse, p. 41.

4 See Devreesse, pp. 58; 94.

V.[1] This may represent "Andegavensis" and may have been written on the manuscript as an indication of its provenance after its inclusion in the papal library.[2] Second, the descriptions of nineteen of the thirty three Greek manuscripts listed in the inventory of the papal library in 1311 contain the note "And."[3] To date only three manuscripts bearing this abbreviation have been identified, Laurentianus Gr. 28,18, Vaticanus Gr. 1605 and Vaticanus Gr. 276,[4] and of these only one, Laurentianus Gr. 28,18, can be securely identified with an entry of the 1311 inventory.[5] Third, V was probably used for the Latin translations of Hippocratic treatises by Bartholomew of Messina while he worked at the court of Manfred from 1258 to 1266.[6] Therefore, although V cannot be identified on either of the early inventories of the papal library, Recensio Bonifatiana (1295) or Recensio Perusina (1311), there is reason to believe that it was part of the papal collection at that time, not long after the 13th c. upheavals in Sicily.[7]

V contains three hands. There is a change of hand on fol. 149ʳ, l. 25 and again on fol. 150ʳ, l. 13 where a third hand appears which completes the manuscript through fol. 207ᵛ.[8] That V is not a copy of a single collection of Hip-

1 See Bagliani, photograph opposite p. 40.

2 In support of "And." = "Andegavensis" see Canart, p. 149 n. 113; G. Derenzini, All'origine della tradizione di opere scientifiche classiche: vicende di testi e di codici tra Bisanzio e Palermo, Physis 18, 1976, pp. 97–100; A. Pelzer, Note, Antiquité Classique 7, 1938, pp. 268–270; A. Rome, Un manuscrit de la bibliothèque de Boniface VIII, Antiquité Classique 7, 1938, pp. 261–268; A. Cappelli, Dizionario di abbreviature latine ed italiane, 6th ed., Milan, 1979, which gives "Andegavensis" as the meaning of "And." with reference to the 15th c. For other interpretations of "And." see Ehrle, pp. 95–96 n. 356 where "And." is taken as an inept abbreviation of "antiquum"; Mercati and Franchi de' Cavalieri, p. 365 where it is suggested that "And." refers to a possible early owner of the manuscript, Andreas de Biagio; Bagliani, pp. 60–69 where he notes the close relationship of "And." to the Latin titles given to the Greek manuscripts as an aid to non-Greek reading librarians during the inventory of Boniface in 1295 and suggests that "And." may be the abbreviated name of the translator of the titles. Against this last interpretation is the fact that "And." also appears on the inferior margin of some pages, with no relation to the Latin title.

3 See Ehrle, pp. 95–99.

4 See Irigoin, L'Italie méridionale, p. 55 n. 70.

5 See A. Pelzer, Addenda et emendanda ad F. Ehrle Historiae Bibliothecae Romanorum Pontificum tum Bonifatianae tum Avenionensis vol. I, Rome, 1947, pp. 93–94.

6 See Irigoin, Tradition, p. 2 n. 2 (= p. 4 n. 3); Jouanna, in: CMG I 1,3, pp. 67; 129–130.

7 Supporting this evidence is general bibliographic information of the period. Other scientific works (mathematics, astronomy, physics) are known to have been part of the library of the Norman kings of Sicily (cf. Canart, p. 149; Irigoin, L'Italie méridionale, pp. 54–55). Also, while the provenance of V before its possible Sicilian sojourn is unknown, it is known that the scientific and philosophic renaissance in Byzantium in the ninth and tenth centuries had produced copies of many technical works and also that some such books in Sicily were presents from the emperor of Byzantium to the Norman kings (cf. also C. H. Haskins and D. P. Lockwood, The Sicilian translators of the twelfth century and the first latin version of Ptolemy's Almagest, Harvard Studies in Classical Philology 21, 1910, pp. 75–102). It is not, therefore, surprising that a medical manuscript may have been included in the Norman library.

8 See Lienau, pp. 13–15.

pocratic works but rather composite, from at least two sources, is shown most clearly by its inclusion of the treatise Περὶ ἐπικυήσιος twice, once by the first hand and once by the third, each copied from a different source. Lienau, who first emphasized V's composite character, calls attention also to physical characteristics of the codex which suggest that it initially ended at fol. 150 and to characteristics of the hands which suggest that the hand of Vb is younger than that of Va.

The treatise De capitis vulneribus occupies folios 57^{r}–61^{r} and 63^{v}. V is the only independent complete manuscript of De capitis vulneribus, the others with the entire text being its descendants. A curious feature of V, however, is its inclusion of two fragments of the treatise De aere aquis locis in the text of De capitis vulneribus, p. 92,1 between ἕλκει and πρὸς (see the app. crit. ad loc.). The inclusion of these two fragments of De aere aquis locis in De capitis vulneribus, the treatise immediately preceding it in the codex, as well as their reversal, is convincingly explained by Ilberg on the basis of transposition of folios, by reversal of a doublepage, in a predecessor of V.[1]

Errors in V:

1. Omissions, for example

Most larger omissions are due to homoioteleuton. There are numerous omissions of single words:

p. 62,9 πεφυκυῖαν om. V

p. 66,19 τῇ om. V

p. 66,21 τῇ – ἐν om. V

p. 66,24 καὶ^{II} – 25 ῥωγμήν om. V

p. 68,3 ἔστι δὲ αὐτέων om. V

p. 68,7 μένον om. V

p. 68,14 ἢ μὴ πέφλασται om. V

p. 70,1 καὶ – 3 τρόπος om. V

p. 70,13 τε^{I} – στεναὶ om. V

p. 72,7 εἴτ'^{I} – ἰσχυροτέροισιν om. V

p. 72,12 τοῦ ἀνθρώπου^{II} om. V

p. 74,3 ἀέκοντος – ὅταν^{II} om. V

p. 74,12 καὶ – ὀστέον^{II} om. V

p. 76,26 οὔτε – 27 διαχαλάσῃ om. V

p. 78,5 καὶ – ὀστέον^{II} om. V

p. 84,5 ἀπρίστῳ om. V

p. 84,5 δέ, καὶ om. V

p. 88,25 ἄν om. V

p. 90,20 ὁ om. V

2. Additions, for example

p. 66,12 ante τῷ add. ἐν V

p. 74,14 ante ὀξὺ add. τε καὶ V

1 J. Ilberg, Zur Überlieferungsgeschichte des Hippokrates, Philologus 52, 1894, p. 424.

p. 76,25 post εὐμαρής add. ἤ V
p. 80,19 post ὅστις add. ἂν V
p. 82,1 post ὀστέῳ add. τοῦ βέλεος V
p. 82,2 post ἕδρην[II] add. τοῦ βέλεος V
p. 92,9 ἢν – πρίεις hab. V

3. Transpositions of words, for example

p. 72,9 καὶ[II] – φάναι post σαρκὸς (lin. 10) trsp. V
p. 72,13 τὸ ὀστέον[II] post ὀφθαλμοῖσι (lin. 14) trsp. V
p. 74,15 κίνδυνος post ὀστέον (lin. 16) trsp. V
p. 80,2 τινὸς δεῖται] δεῖται τινὸς V
p. 82,26–84,1 ἐς πρῖσιν ἀφήκει] ἀφίκει ἐς πρίσιν V

4. Wrong readings, for example

p. 62,16 γραμμέων] γραμμάτων V
p. 64,25 ἔνεστιν] ἐστὶν V
p. 64,28 τὸ ὀστέον ἅπαν τὸ ὄπισθεν] τοῦ ὀστέου πᾶν τὸ ὀστέον V
p. 66,10 ἄνευ ῥωγμῆς] τὰ νεῦρα ἀγμῆς V
p. 68,28 ῥωγμήν] φλάσιν V
p. 70,11 στόμα] σχῆμα V
p. 74,20 φλᾷ καὶ ἔσω ἐσφλᾷ] φλάσει εἴσω ἐς κεφαλήν V
p. 76,14 συγκλέπτει] συμβλέπει V
p. 78,15 οὐδ' ἐπιδεῖν] οὐδὲ πιέζειν V
p. 80,31 μάλα τὸ κακόν] μᾶλλον V
p. 86,14 ποιήσειεν] πυήσηται V

Further errors concern: wrong inflectional endings (p. 62,11 τούτῳ] τούτων; p. 64,18 ἀποθνῄσκει] ἀποθνήσκειν; p. 66,8 ἔχῃ] ἔχων; p. 70,15 ἕδρη] ἕδρην; p. 72,24 ἐξελέγχειν] ἐξελέγχοντα), errors in degrees of comparison (p. 64,23 ὀλιγίστῃ] ὀλίγη; p. 82,10 ἰσχυροτέρου] ἰσχυροῦ), wrong word divisions (p. 66,26 ὥστε οὐ] ὀστέου; p. 70,18 ἄλλῃ] ἀλλ' ἤ; p. 76,21 δὴ ἅτε] διά τε; p. 76,23 μένει] μὲν εἰ; p. 88,9 ἅπαν ὠχρὸν] ἀπάνωχρον; p. 90,15 διαπριωτῷ] διαπρίω τῶ), synonym variants (p. 64,29 ἅπαν] πᾶν; p. 80,5 εὐμαρές] εὐχερὲς; p. 84,11 ἴσχει] ἔχει), mistakes related to uncial script (p. 64,2 σηραγγῶδές] σειραιτῶδες; p. 72,17 ἔργου] ἐρίου; p. 84,6 ὑπόπυον] ὑπὸ πύθη; p. 84,30 ἀποστρακωθὲν] ἀπεστρακὸς, ἐν), orthographic mistakes (iotacisms: p. 62,3 σφίσιν] σφῆσιν; p. 72,10 τι] τοι; p. 82,5 ἀφήκειν] ἀφίκειν; p. 82,15 τηκτὸν] τίκτον; p. 88,10 ἐπιλαμβάνει] ἐπιλαμβάνη; p. 90,1 ἔχῃ[I]] ἔχοι; p. 90,3 ἔχῃ] ἔχοι; p. 90,15 ἐπιλελειμμένῳ] ἐπιλεληιμμένω; confusion of ο and ω: p. 88, 10 γίνονται] γίνωνται; p. 92,2 ὀρῶν] ὀρρὸν).

Other peculiarities in V:

Iota adscript

Iota subscript is not used; iota adscript occurs twice: p. 68,18 ῥωγμῆισιν; p. 92,8 τρυπᾷς] τρυπαῖς.

c) The relationship of B to V

B and V share some passages that are the result of early textual corruption. The most striking example occurs in the account of the types of head injury, pp. 66,21–70,19. Both manuscripts agree on the types and numbers of 1 through 4; V omits the description and number of type 5 (p. 70,1–3); neither has a number 6; both have the description and number of type 7 (p. 70,18–19). Although there are differences in the two accounts, it is clear that each derived from an account already corrupted by the loss of the sixth type, a loss that would not have been apparent except for the numbering. B and V share enough such errors to indicate a moderate degree of textual corruption in their common progenitor. There are, however, enough differences in the two manuscripts to suggest that they represent independent branches which derive from this common ancestor (cf. above, pp. 15–17; 19–20).

Errors common to B and V, which originate in a common ancestor:

1. Omissions, for example

p. 68,1 καὶ^{II} non hab. B V
p. 68,5 πάνυ non hab. B V
p. 68,5 αἳ μὲν non hab. B V
p. 68,28 καὶ^{I} non hab. B V
p. 70,5–6 ἕκτος οὗτος τρόπος non hab. B V
p. 72,19 ἢ^{II} non hab. B V
p. 80,13 ἐν τῷ non hab. B V
p. 84,1 ἡ non hab. B V

2. Additions

p. 66,17 ἢ hab. B V
p. 78,7 τε^{I} hab. B V

3. Wrong readings, for example

p. 64,22 ταύτῃ] ταύτην B V
p. 64,31 ἐόντων] ἁπάντων B V
p. 66,16 ἕλκος] βέλος B V
p. 72,9 ἤισαν] εἴησαν B V
p. 72,23 τούτων] τουτ(ε)ω B V
p. 74,3 βουλομένου] βουλόμενος B V
p. 74,6 τιτρώσκῃ] τιτρώσκει B V
p. 76,17 γινομένῃ] γινομένησι B V
p. 82,20 μέλαινα] μέλαν B V
p. 82,22. 26 βάϑος] βάϑους B V

Differing errors in B and V which permit inference of textual corruption in the common ancestor, for example:

1. Additions

p. 62,6 post τούτου hab. τέ B, δ' V
p. 64,32 μειόνων hab. V, μιονος B

2. Wrong readings

p. 64,22 ὑπὸ λεπτοτάτῳ γὰρ] υπο λεπτω τε γαρ B: ὑπολεπτώτεταος V
p. 66,27 ἔστιν αἳ τῶν] ἐστι δε των B: ἔστι δ' αἴτιον V
p. 68,26 ἕδρῃ] ἑδραιηι B: ἑδρέη V
p. 72,20 γε ἐόντος] τεοντος B: τὲ ἐόντος V
p. 74,6 ἀσθενέστερον] ἀσθενεστερος B: ἀσθενεστέρως V
p. 74,24. 26 φλᾷ τε] φλεται B: φλᾶται V
p. 76,17 τὸ πολὺ τῇ] τόπου αυτησιν B: τὸ πουλὺ αὕτη V
p. 80,3 καὶ ὅταν] και ον ἀν B: κακὸν ἂν V

All in all, B offers the more reliable text, but V in some individual instances retains the correct reading. In most cases in which B and V differ from one another the reading of B has been accepted.

d) The descendants of B

1. Parisinus Gr. 2248

N Parisinus Gr. 2248 (= N) is a large 16th c. paper codex of 670 folios. The three introductory poems of B occur on folios $15^{r}-17^{v}$. A fourth poem has been added to N, on fol. 1^{rv} (the index occupies the pages between this poem and the first of the other poems), acknowledging that Lorenzo de' Medici was responsible for the acquisition of B.[1] The hand throughout the manuscript is clear and heavy with considerable discoloration of the paper around each character, a sort of dark halo. This spreading of or reaction to the ink disappears after fol. 113. From the top of fol. 114, although the hand is the same, the characters are distinct, due presumably either to a difference in ink, writing instrument or paper. Around fol. 135 the blurring of the characters recurs and persists through the rest of the text. Following the text and occupying folios 556– 670 are illustrations of treatment (manipulation, reduction, and bandages)[2] which are attributed to the painter John of Santorini.[3]

Schöne provides the most complete account of the provenance of N.[4] In 1534 Pope Clement VII, né Giulio de' Medici, had B brought to Rome where he entrusted it for revision to Janus Lascaris who had bought it for Lorenzo de' Medici 42 years before. Lascaris undertook the revision; however, Lascaris died in 1535, probably leaving his emendations of B in the form of loose

1 Lascaris is not mentioned in the poem, and this fact suggested to Schöne, p. XXI, that its author was Lascaris.
2 Those illustrations pertaining to the head are found on folios 609–612; 622–635; 645–649; 660–665.
3 See Schöne, p. XIX (no. 114).
4 Schöne, pp. XVII–XXI.

manuscript notes, which were later incorporated in a copy of B, this copy being codex N.

The treatise De capitis vulneribus is located on folios 105^{v}–116^{v}. It ends at the point where passages of De aere aquis locis are inserted in the manuscript V. It is followed by Mochlikon.

The text of De capitis vulneribus in this manuscript must be considered in two sections, the first from the beginning through p. 84,25, where the text of this treatise in B breaks off, and the second from that point to the end. For the last section the scribe of N had to use an exemplar of another tradition. Concerning the first section, N is an essentially faithful copy of the text that survives in B.

The most impressive similarities between N and B are the omissions. All the omissions of B occur as well in N – with the exception of the passages missing in the text of B but supplied in the margin by B^{2} (pp. 66,1–2; 82,4. 11) –, e.g.:

p. 68,26 τῇ τε ῥωγμῇ om. BN
p. 72,1 καὶ – 2 ἐσφλασθέντα om. BN
p. 78,9 ἢ – δεξάμενος om. BN
p. 80,13 ἣν – 14 ἐπιλαμβάνει om. BN

In general, the forms and the readings of B are retained, e.g.:

p. 62,5 τὸ V: αὐτέου BN
p. 62,26 μαλθακώτερον] μαλθακότατον B: μαλθακώτατον N
p. 64,6 ἔνεστι δ'] ἔνεστιν BN: ἔνι δ' V
p. 64,22 ὑπὸ λεπτοτάτῳ γὰρ] υπο λεπτω τε γαρ BN: ὑπολεπτώτεταος V
p. 66,11 δὲ γίνονται V: δ' ἐπιγίνονται BN
p. 66,12 ἐκ τουτέων V: εξ ων BN
p. 66,22; 68,26 προσγενέσθαι] προσγίγνεσθαι BN
p. 72,11 ἀπόπροσθεν] ἀποπρισθὲν BN
p. 76,13 ἔνεστιν ἐν] ἔνεστι μὲν BN
p. 76,24 διαχάλασίς] διαχαλασιης B: διὰ χαλασίης N
p. 80,17 ὅση ἂν δοκῇ] οκοσηι ην δοκεηι B: ὅκως ᾗ, ἣν δοκέῃ N
p. 80,30 ἐσφλωμένης] εσφαλωμενης B: ἐσφαλυμένης N

There are also attempts to improve readings, including changes in spelling, e.g.:

p. 62,3 σφίσιν] φησὶν B N in textu, οἶμαι, φύσιν N in marg.
p. 62,8 πεφυκοῖαν B: πεφυκυῖαν N
p. 62,16 γραμμαιων B: γραμμέων N
p. 62,23 ἡ V: ἣν B: ᾗ ἡ N
p. 64,2 μαλθακότατον B: μαλθακώτατον N
p. 64,15 φλᾶται τε V: φλατεται B: φλᾶται N
p. 66,23 περ V: τερ B: τε N
p. 66,25 εἴδεαι B: ἰδέαι N
p. 68,1 πόνων] ποιεων B: ποίεον in textu, ἴσως πύελον in marg. N
p. 76,8 σημεια B: σημήια N

p. 76,25 οὔτε ἀπὸ] ουτε η απο B: οὔτε εἰ ἀπὸ N: οὔτε ὑπὸ V
p. 80,3 καὶ ὅταν] και ον ἀν B: καὶ ἂν N: κακὸν ἂν V
p. 84,22 μυδᾷ τε] μυδαι τε B: μύδηται N: μηδύη τὲ V
p. 84,22 ξαινηται B: ξηραίνηται N

Errors peculiar to N are the following:

1. Addition

p. 64,1 post πυκνὸν add. δὲ N

2. Wrong readings, e.g.

p. 70,10 κυκλοτερής] κυκλωτέρη N
p. 74,11 ἐσπίπτοντα] ἐπιπίπτοντα N
p. 76,11 κατ' αὐτὰς] κατὰ ταύτας N
p. 82,13 κατέπεσεν] ἔπεσε N

To the text of De capitis vulneribus derived from B there are three marginalia written by the scribe himself:

p. 62,3 σφίσιν] φησὶν in textu, οἶμαι, φύσιν in marg. N
p. 68,1 πόνων] ποίεον in textu, ἴσως πύελον in marg. N
p. 84,22 ξαίνηται] ξηραίνηται in textu, γρ' ἐξαίρηται[1] in marg. N

For the determination of the source from which N took the second segment of the work, it is important to note that the peculiarities of N in this segment do not agree with those of only one manuscript. On the other hand, there are several passages in which N and the Aldine edition share readings peculiar to themselves:

p. 86,10 δ' ἐκ] δὲ ἐκ Ald. N
p. 86,19 σηραγγώδεα] σηραιτώδεα V: οὐ σκληρώδεα Ho^2: οὔτε σκληρώδεα Ald. N
p. 86,35 τάδε] τόδε Ald. N
p. 88,13 τὰ] τὸ V: τὰ Ald. N
p. 90,32 τὸν πρίονα] τὴν πρίονα V: τὸν πρίονα Ald. N

Also, the Aldine is the first text from which the scribe of N could have learned that the text of De capitis vulneribus had been disrupted by incorporation of extraneous material (the passages from De aere aquis locis), a fact that led him to end the text at τῷ ἕλκει (p. 92,1).

The Froben edition as a possible source for N is eliminated since, on the one hand, it shares only three of the above mentioned agreements between the Aldine and N (pp. 86,10; 88,13; 90,32), and, on the other hand, it has readings which are not found in N:

p. 84,30 ἀποστρακωθὲν] ἀπεστρακὸς, ἐν V Ald. N: ἀποστρακὸς, ἐν Frob.
p. 86,19 σηραγγώδεα] σηραιτώδεα V: οὔτε σκληρώδεα Ald. N: οὔτε σηραγγώδεα Frob.
p. 88,19 καπυρὸν V Ald. N: εὔπριστον Frob.

[1] See below, p. 25 n. 1.

p. 90,10 τελευτῶσά πη V Ald. N: τελευταῖον σάπη Frob.
p. 90,15 διαπριωτῷ] διαπρίω τῶ V Ald. N: διαπριωτῷ Frob.
p. 90,33 πάχιστον (-υστον Ald.) V Ald. N: παχύτατον Frob.

Differences between the texts of N and the Aldine do not necessarily argue against the Aldine as a source for this part of N. Six readings are those of V; they may represent corrections of errors in the Aldine rather than direct use of V or its apographs (p. 88,8 τηνικαῦται Ald.: τηνικαῦτα V N; p. 88,20 εὔξηστον Ald.: εὔξυστον V N; p. 90,10 πολὴν χρόνον Ald.: πουλὺν χρόνον V N; p. 90,16 λοιπόμενον Ald.: λειπόμενον V N; p. 90,32 ὅπῃ] ὅτη Ald.: ὅπη V N; p. 90,33 δοκέη Ald.: δοκέει V N). Other differences consist first of corrections of the transmitted text (p. 84,29 ξηραίνοιτο V Ald.: ξηραίνοι τὸ N; p. 86,1 ἀφίεται V Ald.: ἀφί^{στα}εται N; p. 88,5 ῥέοι V Ald.: ῥέει N; p. 88,17 ἐννοίης V Ald.: ἐννοοίης N; p. 90,20 ὁ add. N) and secondly of errors peculiar to N (p. 86,11 τοῦ ὀστέου^{II} om. N; p. 88,11 ἐπ' – 13 τῷ om. N; p. 90,1 ἔχῃ^{II}] ἔχοι N; p. 90,15 ἐπιλελειμμένῳ] ἐπιλεληημμένω V Ald.: ἐπελελη$^{\mu}$σμένῳ N; p. 90,31 ᾗ τὸ τρῶμα, ᾗ] ἣ τὸ τρῶμα N).

Accordingly, N from the beginning of the text up to p. 84,25 τῷ ὀ(στέῳ) is an accurate copy of B with a few changes, which are probably the emendations of Lascaris. From p. 84,25 to p. 92,1 ἕλκει N represents the V-tradition[1], with the Aldine as its principal source.

2. Parisinus Gr. 2247

Parisinus Gr. 2247 (= M) is a large 16th c. paper manuscript of 415 pages. On the second blank at the front of the codex a notice in the hand of the scribe informs the reader that the manuscript contains the collection of surgical treatises made by Nicetas. M

The three introductory poems of B occur in M on folios 10^{v}–12^{r}; however, the poem that pays tribute to Lorenzo de' Medici in N is not included in M. Instead, on fol. 12^{r}, there is a brief elegy by Lascaris, praising John of Santorini, the illustrator of N. The script of M is a large and clear minuscule. Each treatise begins with a decorated capital. The illustrations at the end of the codex, similar to those of N but finer, are attributed to the painter Francesco Primaticcio. This manuscript was written by the calligrapher Christophe Auer who worked in Rome from 1541 to 1548. From catalogue evidence, one can conclude that M was in Fontainebleau before 1546.[2]

The fact that M is a copy of N[3] is also shown by the treatise De capitis vulneribus which is contained on folia 71^{v}–79^{v} and which ends, as in N, at the place where the passages from De aere aquis locis are inserted in V.

M reproduces the text of N with all its peculiarities, e.g.:

1 Traces of this tradition can also be found in the text immediately preceding: p. 84,5 ἀπρίστῳ et δέ, καὶ om. V Ald. N; p. 84,8 φλεγμαίνῃ τε] φλεγμαίνηται V Ald. N; p. 84, 22 ξαίνηται] ἐξαίρηται V Ald.: γρ' ἐξαίρηται in marg. N.

2 See Schöne, pp. XVIII; XXI–XXII.

3 See Schöne, pp. XXI–XXII.

1. Omissions

p. 86,11 τοῦ ὀστέου^{II} om. NM
p. 88,11 ἐπ' – 13 τῷ om. NM

2. Addition

p. 64,1 post πυκνὸν add. δὲ NM

3. Wrong readings, for example

p. 74,11 ἐσπίπτοντα] ἐπιπίπτοντα NM
p. 76,24 διαχάλασίς] διαχαλασιης B: διὰ χαλασίης NM
p. 82,13 κατέπεσεν] ἔπεσε NM
p. 90,31 ᾗ τὸ τρῶμα, ᾗ] ἡ τὸ τρῶμα NM

4. Corrections

p. 84,29 ξηραίνοι τὸ NM: ξηραίνοιτο V Ald.
p. 86,1 ἀφίσταται] ἀφί^(στα)εται NM

M also shows itself a true copy of N in its repetition of the three marginalia (see above, p. 24).

e) The descendants of V

Four of the younger manuscripts, Palatinus Gr. 192, Monacensis Gr. 71, Parisinus Gr. 2146, and Holkhamensis Gr. 92, depend directly on the text of V.[1]

1. Palatinus Gr. 192

P Palatinus Gr. 192 (= P) is a 15th c. paper manuscript, containing on 180 folios, in two columns per folio, the same collection of Hippocratic treatises as V, in the same order as V through Κατ' ἰητρεῖον, and then in a different order.[2] An index, in the hand of the scribe and on the first folio along with the first work, Ὅρκος, and the beginning of Νόμος, is identical to that of V, listing 62 works.[3] An owner's note, now attached to the bottom of fol. 180^{v}, states: "Andreae de Biago (sic) – Questo libro e di francesco di nicholaio bili-

1 The texts of other Hippocratic treatises (De corde, De carn., De superf., De aere aquis locis) confirm that these manuscripts are copies of V; see F. C. Unger, Liber Hippocraticus Περὶ καρδίης, Mnemosyne 51, 1923, pp. 4; 6; Schubring, pp. XII–XIV; Lienau, p. 20; Diller, in: CMG I 1,2, pp. 7–8.

2 See Ilberg, Überlieferung, pp. 447–448 for a list of the contents. Giving the sequence of the treatises, Ilberg points out that Περὶ ἐπικυήσιος occurs just once.

3 There are two additions in another hand. The first addition, following Προγνωστικόν, is Περὶ πτισάνης (the title of this work, on fol. 13^{v}, is Πρὸς τὰς Κνιδίας γνώμας ἢ περὶ πτισάνης). This treatise occurs in the same location in V and is also missing in the index to V. The second addition is Περὶ ἰητροῦ following Κατ' ἰητρίον (sic), indicating the point at which the index and the actual order deviate.

otti da firenze lo quale tiene messer giovanni aurispa dalo detto francesco in soma di piu altri libri; e pero io francesco sopradetto ho fatto questi versi di mia di mia (sic) propria mano questo di VI di Luglio 1457 in Roma."[1] On a front blank is another manuscript note, "Iannocii Manetti Carte 180. Tractatus 62 hippocratis"[2], and beneath this a bookplate stating, "Sum de Bibliotheca, quam Heidelberga capta, Spolium fecit, et P. M. Gregorio XV trophaeum misit Maximilianus Utriusque Bavariae Dux etc. S. R. I. Archidapifer et Princeps Elector. Anno Christi 1623."[3] The exact odyssey of P leading to its inclusion in the Palatine Library is not known. Giovanni Aurispa (1376–1459) was one of Renaissance Italy's most avid book collectors.[4] Cornarius in his preface to the 1538 Froben edition of Hippocrates lists, among the manuscripts he consulted in its preparation, one codex from the library of Ioannes Dalburg.[5] The library of Dalburg went to enlarge the Palatine Library.[6] Rivier postulates, without any stated basis, that the manuscript mentioned by Cornarius was P.[7] The facts are compatible; however, without proof that P was part of Dalburg's library the identification must remain tentative.

De capitis vulneribus is contained on folios 64rb to 68rb and 70va, the sections of De aere aquis locis occupying the hiatus. It is followed by Περὶ ἄρθρων ἐμβολῆς which begins on a separate folio.[8] The few corrections which occur in De capitis vulneribus appear to be in the hand of the scribe. There are no marginalia.

2. Monacensis Gr. 71

Monacensis Gr. 71 (= Mo) is a 15th c. paper manuscript on 406 folios Mo
containing, in order, Galen's Hippocratic Lexicon, abridged, Soranus' Life of Hippocrates and a large number of Hippocratic works.[9] It is the work of two scribes, one responsible for folios 1 through 179^{v} and 370^{r} through 406^{r}, the

1 Stevenson, p. 97, says of this note: "Ad calcem codicis fragmentum folii quod integrum olim in fronte positum erat." Stevenson, pp. 90 and 93, also reports owners' notes, identical except for the repetition, on two other Palatine mss., Palat. Gr. 170 and Palat. Gr. 176.

2 Iannotius Manetti was the owner of a large number of mss. now in the Palatine collection at the Vatican. See Stevenson, p. 302.

3 Maximilian's Catholic forces took Heidelberg in September, 1622. The Church of the Holy Spirit was turned over to the Jesuits, and the Palatine Library, which was housed in the church, was sent to Rome.

4 Dizionario Biografico degli Italiani, Istituto della Enciclopedia Italiana, Rome, 1962, vol. 4, pp. 593–595. This article, p. 594, quotes Aurispa's own description of his obsession.

5 Allgemeine Deutsche Biographie, Berlin, 1968, vol. 4, pp. 702–703, describes Johann von Dalburg, born 1455, died 1503, Bishop of Worms and Chancellor of the University of Heidelberg, as a scholar who had studied in Italy and from that time became an educator with a strong interest in Greek literature and an avid collector of manuscripts.

6 See Stevenson, pp. XXIII–XXIV.

7 Rivier, p. 155 n. 4.

8 The index says that De capitis vulneribus is preceded by Περὶ ἄρθρων and followed by Περὶ ἀέρων τόπων ὑδάτων.

9 Cf. Ilberg, Überlieferung, pp. 460–461; Mondrain, pp. 201–214.

other for folios 180^r through 369^v.[1] However, the first scribe has contributed words, lines, even an entire page to the work of the second, without loss of continuity or repetition. Therefore Mondrain is certainly correct in regarding the scribes as contemporary and the first as the mentor and reviser of the second. The first scribe remains anonymous; the second, however, has been identified by Mondrain as a pupil of George Gemiste Plethon at Mistra, one Demetrios Raoul Kabakes, who was in Rome from 1466. On the basis of the watermarks of two other manuscripts due to Kabakes, Monacenses Gr. 237 and 336, she estimates that Mo was most likely copied during the decade 1470–1480.[2]

According to a presentation inscription (fol. 1), dated 1577, Mo belonged to Adolphus Occo I[3] (1447–1503), a physician and a scholar of Greek in Augsburg, grandfather of the author of the inscription, Adolphus Occo III (1524–1606), also a physician and humanist of Augsburg, who dedicated the manuscript to Albert, Duke of Bavaria.[4]

The text in Mo combines different textual traditions. The majority of the treatises are derived from Parisinus Gr. 2140 (= I; 12th/13th c.), which, in turn, relies on Marcianus Gr. 269 (= M; 10th c.). But those treatises contained in Mo and not descended from I, depend instead on V.[5]

De capitis vulneribus is contained on folios 398^r to 402^v and 406^r, the hiatus containing the sections of De aere aquis locis as in V. De capitis vulneribus is the last treatise in the codex and was copied by the first scribe. Corrections and marginalia are few and appear, for the most part, to be in the hand of the scribe.

3. Parisinus Gr. 2146

C Parisinus Gr. 2146 (= C) is a paper manuscript of the 16th c., containing on 352 folios the index of V and a large number of Hippocratic treatises. The scribe was Constantine Mesobotes, a copyist active in Padua and other northern Italian cities in the first half of the 16th c.[6] The entire manuscript, except for some corrections, is written in the same hand. On the last page is written ἱπποκράτους πάντα τὰ εὑρισμένα No 47. The number 47 was given the

1 Mondrain, p. 203, has identified two other hands which appear sporadically in the section written by the second scribe.

2 See Mondrain, pp. 202–203.

3 Mondrain, p. 211, has identified manuscript notes of A. Occo I in Mo in the margins of De morbo sacro.

4 In his preface to the 1538 Froben edition of Hippocrates Cornarius mentions three manuscripts he consulted (see below, p. 41). One of them can probably be identified with Mo. On the last page of this manuscript is written "1531", in a hand different from either of the scribes. This hand has not been firmly identified as that of Cornarius. However, Mondrain, pp. 212–213, suggests the possibility: "la date de 1531 ... me semble correspondre au moment où Cornarius avait obtenu le manuscrit d'Occo".

5 See Schubring, p. XIII.

6 Gamillscheg and Harlfinger, II A, p. 123.

manuscript while it was in the collection of Cardinal Ridolfi[1] whose library was bought by Pietro Strozzi, then passed, in part, to Catherine de' Medici, and through her entered the French Royal Library in 1599.[2]

De capitis vulneribus is located on folios 92^{v} to 99^{r} and 103^{v}. The usual sections of De aere aquis locis occupy the hiatus. There are numerous corrections, usually written superscript, some perhaps in the hand of the scribe. The marginalia are almost all words or passages omitted from the text and supplied in very small letters.

4. Holkhamensis Gr. 92

Holkhamensis Gr. 92 (formerly 282) (= Ho) is a 16th c. paper manuscript, **Ho** copied by Constantine Mesobotes, the scribe responsible as well for C.[3] It contains, on II + 489 leaves, 28 Hippocratic treatises preceded by Galen's Hippocratic Lexicon. In 1639 it was in Padua, owned by the library of S. Giovanni in Verdara.[4]

De capitis vulneribus is located on folios 168^{r} to 178^{v} and 186^{rv}. Between the body of De capitis vulneribus and its short closing passage occur the usual sections of De aere aquis locis. The hand throughout is identical with that of C (recumbent ε's, low δ's, open ϑ's). There is also a distinctive form of the marginal abbreviation, Ση, for σημείωσαι, found occasionally in both manuscripts. Further similarities of Ho and C are frequent use of ν moveable and the large number of omissions (see below, p. 31).[5] Some corrections in Ho appear to be in the hand of the scribe, e.g. $υ^{I}$ of ἀπορρυγνύμενόν changed to η (p. 68,19), ἄρης changed to εὕρης (p. 72,15). However, most of the corrections are by one or more other hands (= Ho^{2}), characterized by crude and **Ho^{2}** awkward Greek letters, quite different from those of the original scribe (see below, p. 32).

5. The relationship of P, Mo, C, Ho to V

On the basis of shared peculiarities the manuscripts P, Mo, C and Ho prove to be copies of V. On p. 92,1, the same insertion of passages from De aere aquis locis as in V is to be found in these manuscripts. Also peculiarities of orthography and accentuation conform to those of V.

1 See Rivier, p. 139 n. 2.

2 See H. Omont, Inventaire sommaire des manuscrits grecs de la Bibliothèque Nationale, vol. II, Paris, 1888, p. XXVI.

3 See Gamillscheg and Harlfinger, I A, pp. 124–125; Alexanderson, p. 78; H. Diller, Die Überlieferung der hippokratischen Schrift Περὶ ἀέρων ὑδάτων τόπων, Leipzig, 1932 (Philologus Suppl. 23,3), p. 10.

4 See R. Barbour, Summary description of the Greek manuscripts from the library at Holkham Hall, Bodleian Library Record VI, no. 5, 1960, p. 609.

5 However, the omissions do not coincide, and, except for the shared ἐπὶ παλαιότερον (p. 68,24), the readings that deviate from V are peculiar to each, indicating that Mesobotes used V as the model independently for both C and Ho.

Further similarities are found in this group of manuscripts: all the omissions of passages or single words which are found in V (e.g.: p. 66,24 καὶ^{II} – 25 ῥωγμήν; p. 68,7 μένον; p. 70,1 καὶ – 3 τρόπος; p. 72,7 εἴτ'^{I} – ἰσχυροτέροισιν; p. 84,5 ἀπρίστῳ), additions to the text (e.g.: p. 74,14 ante ὀξὺ add. τε καὶ; p. 80,19 post ὅστις add. ἂν; p. 82,1 post ὀστέῳ add. τοῦ βέλεος), transposition of words (e.g.: p. 72,9 καὶ^{II} – φάναι post σαρκὸς (lin. 10) trsp.; p. 80,2 τινὸς δεῖται] δεῖται τινὸς), wrong readings (e.g.: p. 64,2 σηραγγῶδές] σειραιτῶδες; p. 66,10 ἄνευ ῥωγμῆς] τὰ νεῦρα ἀγμῆς; p. 72,17 ἔργου] ἐρίου; p. 76,14 συγκλέπτει] συμβλέπει; p. 80,17 τομήν] τολίην).

In some places these manuscripts have corrected or tried to correct clearly recognizable errors of the exemplar, at times concurring, at times differing:

p. 64,12 δὴ ὅτι] διότ V: διότι P Mo C Ho
p. 66,12 θάνανατος V: θάνατος P Mo C Ho
p. 86,8 κινδυνεύειν] κινδεύειν V C: κιν$^{\text{//}}$δεύειν P: κινδ^{ιν}εύειν Mo: κινδυνεύειν Ho
p. 64,22 ὑπὸ λεπτοτάτῳ γὰρ] ὑπολεπτώτεταος V P Ho: ὑπολεπτώτατος Mo: ὑπὸ λεπτώτητος C
p. 64,18 ἀποθνήσκειν V P Mo: ἀποθνήσκει C: ἀποθνήσκε^{ει}ιν Ho
p. 68,24 ἐπιπολαιότερον] ἐπὶ πολαιότερον V P Mo: ἐπὶ παλαιότερον C Ho
p. 88,9 ἅπαν ὠχρὸν] ἀπάνωχρον V P Mo: ἐπάνωχρον C: ἐπάνοχρον Ho

Apart from these similarities all four manuscripts show sufficient peculiarities to prove that, independent from one another, they go back to V.

Errors in P, for example:

1. Omissions

p. 66,14 τοῦ om. P
p. 76,11 τὰς om. P

2. Wrong readings

p. 66,19 τοσούσδε] τουσούδε P
p. 70,7 προσγένηται] προσγίνηται V: προσγίγνηται P
p. 72,18–19 εἰ ... ἢ^{I}] ἢ ... εἰ P
p. 80,10 ἔτι] ἔστι P

Corrections in P:

p. 72,4 διακοπὴ] διαπὴ V: δια^{κο}πή P
p. 90,15 διαπρίω τῶ V: διαπριωτῶ P

Errors in Mo[1]:

Wrong readings

p. 66,3 παχύτητα] ταχύτητα Mo
p. 90,33 πάχιστον] τάχιστον Mo

1 Mo is a very accurate copy of V.

Errors in C:

1. Omissions, most due to homoioteleuton,[1] for example

p. 68,2 τῶν – 3 ῥήγνυνται om. C
p. 70,4 τῇ – 6 τῷ om. C
p. 72,27 ἅπερ – 29 ὀστέον om. C
p. 84,16 ὑποπύους – 17 ἕλκος om. C
p. 84,18 βλαστούσης – 19 ἕλκος om. C
p. 84,26 ἀφίσταται – 27 ὀστέου om. C
p. 86,19 διὰ – 20 στερεά om. C
p. 86,27 ἢ – πέφλασται[II] om. C
p. 88,15 ἢ – 16 ταῦτα om. C

2. Wrong readings, for example

p. 62,18 μακρῇσι bis scr. C
p. 64,12 οὕτως ταῦτα] ταῦτα οὕτω C
p. 64,24 κροτάφους] κροτάφας C
p. 64,25 κίνησις] κλίνησις C
p. 68,14 πέφλασται[I]] πέφλαται C
p. 72,4 διακοπὴ] διαπή V: διαπτὰ C
p. 74,5 βέλος] σκέλος C
p. 74,29 φλασθείσας] σφλασθείσας C

Correction in C:

p. 88,10 γίνωνται V: γίνονται C

Errors in Ho:

1. Omissions, in part due to homoioteleuton

p. 62,25 τοῦ[II] om. Ho
p. 64,22 ὀστέῳ[I] om. Ho, in marg. add. Ho[2]
p. 66,12 ὁ om. Ho
p. 68,8 τρόπος om. Ho
p. 68,10 διὰ – 11 καὶ[II] om. Ho
p. 68,16 τε om. Ho
p. 70,4 ἐν[II] om. Ho, supra lin. add. Ho[2]
p. 72,9 τὸ[II] om. Ho
p. 78,8 ὁ om. Ho
p. 84,10 καὶ[II] – σφυγμὸν om. Ho
p. 84,11 κακὰ om. Ho
p. 84,22 ὑγρὴ om. Ho

2. Addition

p. 80,3 ante τὸ add. μὲν Ho

[1] These omissions are supplied in very small letters in the inner margins. They may possibly be in the hand of Mesobotes, but are too small and cramped to allow certain identification.

3. Wrong readings

p. 64,20 ἐγκέφαλος] ἐγγέφαλος Ho
p. 66,15 τύχοι] τύχη Ho
p. 70,15 μένῃ] μένει Ho
p. 72,6 ἔχει] ἔχη Ho
p. 72,25 ἑωυτῷ] ἑαυτῶ V: αὐτῶ Ho
p. 78,27 τι σίνος] τί σινὸς V: τὸ σίνος Ho
p. 80,22 μάζῃ] μάζην Ho
p. 80,30 κεφαλῆς] φαλῆς Ho

Corrections or attempted corrections in Ho:

p. 86,19 σηραγγώδεα] σηραιτώδεα V: σκληραιτώδεα Ho
p. 88,10 ἐπιλαμβάνη V: ἐπιλαμβάνει Ho

Corrections or attempted corrections in later hands in Ho (= Ho²), in part in accord with the readings of B:

p. 64,7 σκληρότητος ... μαλθακότητος ... κοιλότητος recte Ho: σκληρότητι ... μαλθακότητι ... κοιλότητι Ho²
p. 64,22 ὑπὸ λεπτοτάτῳ γὰρ] υπο λεπτω τε γαρ B: ὑπολεπτώτεταος Ho: ὑπολεπτοτάτω γὰρ Ho²
p. 64,22 ταύτην Ho: ταύτη B³ Ho²
p. 64,28 τὸ^I – ὄπισθεν] τοῦ ὀστέου πᾶν τὸ ὀστέον Ho: τοῦ ὀστέου παντὸς τὸ ὀστέον Ho²
p. 66,17 ἐοῦσαι] οὖσαι ἢ Ho: ἢ del. Ho²
p. 72,4 διακοπὴ] διαπὴ Ho: διακοπὴ B Ho²
p. 74,16 κατ' ἐναντίον Ho: κατ' ἀντίον B Ho²
p. 78,2 ῥωμοειδέες Ho: ῥωγμοειδέες B Ho²
p. 78,10 ἀποχωρῆσαι τὰ Ho: ἀποχωρήσαντα B Ho²
p. 78,14 τείνειν Ho: τέγγειν B Ho²
p. 78,20 ἐπιρροῆς Ho: ἐπιρροήν B Ho²
p. 80,16 ἐπέχει Ho: εἴ τι ἔχει B Ho²
p. 80,22 δὲ μάσσειν recte Ho: διαμάσσειν Ho²
p. 80,22 ἕψειν δὲ] ἢ ἕψειν δὲ Ho: δὲ del. Ho²
p. 82,15 τὸ τηκτὸν] τὸ τίκτον Ho: τήκων Ho²
p. 82,15 δεύσαντα] δεύσαντι Ho: δεύσας τι Ho²
p. 82,17 post ἀπολύσας add. καὶ Ho²
p. 82,22 μέλαιναν del. Ho²
p. 84,6 ὑπὸ πύθη Ho: ὑπόπυον B Ho²
p. 86,13 διαπύθη Ho: διάπυον Ho²
p. 86,14 ποιήσειεν] πυήσηται Ho: ποιήσηται Ho²
p. 86,19 σηραγγώδεα] σκληραιτώδεα Ho: οὐ σκληρώδεα Ho²
p. 88,9 ἅπαν ὠχρὸν] ἐπάνοχρον Ho: ἔπωχρον Ho²
p. 88,17 εἰ add. Ho²
p. 92,9 ἣν – πρίεις del. Ho²

The great number of corrections in Ho point to the fact that this manuscript played a role in connection with the printing of the Aldine edition (see below, pp. 39–41).

f) Parisinus Gr. 2255 and its printed source

E

Parisinus Gr. 2255 (= E) is a paper manuscript of 397 folios that up to fol. 366^{v} is of the 15th century.[1] This part of E together with its fellow manuscript, Parisinus Gr. 2254, contains the Hippocratic treatises of the collectio Marciana. The text of E, to fol. 366^{v}, is in one hand with corrections and marginal notes in other hands. The following fourteen treatises of the V-tradition beginning in the middle of fol. 366^{v} have been added in order to supplement the collectio Marciana. Their text is in a very small clear hand, often with minimal separation between treatises. The impression, after the normal-sized script and elaborate initials of the body of the manuscript, is of miniturization and compression to accomodate on as few pages as possible those Hippocratic treatises not in the collectio Marciana. Other texts of this group, to which De capitis vulneribus belongs, have been proven to have been copied from the Froben edition of 1538.[2]

The first description of E occurs in the catalogues of the library of Fontainebleau, compiled by Ange Vergèce and Constantine Palaeocappa between 1549 and 1552.[3] The description leaves no doubt that the manuscript described was E and states specifically that the number of treatises it contained at that time was 39, i.e. the 14 treatises at the back had been added.[4] That means that the addition of this series of texts to E must have taken place between 1538 and 1552.

The treatise De capitis vulneribus occupies folios 389^{v} to 393^{r}. It concludes with the phrase that precedes the sections of De aere aquis locis which are incorporated in De capitis vulneribus in the manuscript V, ξυμφέρειν τῷ ἕλκει (p. 92,1), followed by a phrase supplied by the scribe of the small hand, so that the final sentence ends, ὡς ἂν δοκέῃ ξυμφέρειν τῷ ἕλκει. καὶ ἐπιμελεῖσθαι μή τι ἐπικίνδυνον ξυμβῇ. The end of De capitis vulneribus, p. 92,3 Καὶ – 8 γέγραπται, introduced in the Aldine and Froben editions by the title, Καὶ τάδε τὰ τελευταῖα ὑπό τινος προσγεγράφθαι δῆλον ἐστίν, has been omitted in E. The sections of De aere aquis locis associated with De capitis vulneribus have been treated as a separate treatise, titled Ἱπποκράτους περὶ προγνώσεως ἐτῶν· οἱ δὲ, τινὸς ἄλλου παλαιοῦ. The first few sentences of these passages, ὅτι – ἔχει (CMG I 1,2, p. 46,5–16) have been switched to the

1 See Rivier, p. 106 n. 1.

2 See Diller, in: CMG I 1,2, pp. 12–22; id., Nochmals: Überlieferung und Text der Schrift von der Umwelt, in: Festschrift Ernst Kapp, Hamburg, 1958, p. 31 n. 2; U. Fleischer, Untersuchungen zu den pseudohippokratischen Schriften Παραγγελίαι, Περὶ ἰητροῦ und Περὶ εὐσχημοσύνης, Berlin, 1939 (Neue Deutsche Forschungen, Abt. Klassische Philologie 10), pp. 51–53; K. Schubring, Untersuchungen zur Überlieferungsgeschichte der hippokratischen Schrift De locis in homine, Berlin, 1941 (Neue Deutsche Forschungen, Abt. Klassische Philologie 12), p. 39; Alexanderson, pp. 82–83.

3 For dates, see Omont, p. IX n. 1.

4 See Omont, pp. 101–102; 334–335.

end, following πρὸς τὸ (τὸν E) γινόμενον ὁρῶν (ὀρρὸν E; p. 92,2), and the sentence περὶ – ὑγιηρόν (CMG I 1,2, p. 46,16–18) has been rearranged to begin the "new treatise".

The evidence supplied by De capitis vulneribus supports the premise that the Froben edition was the source for the treatises of the V-tradition in E. For the Froben is the only witness to readings otherwise peculiar to E:

p. 64,9 post λεπτότητι add. οὕτως Frob.E
p. 70,19 ἕβδομος] πέμπτος Frob.E
p. 80,15–16 ὀστέου ... ἐψιλωμένου] ὀστέων ... ἐψιλωμένων Frob.E
p. 80,28 αὖτις] αὖθις Frob.E
p. 82,20 μέλαν ἐὸν Frob.E: μελανεον B: μελάνεον V Ald.
p. 84,30 ἀποστρακωθὲν] ἀποστρακὸς, ἐν Frob.E: ἀπεστρακὸς, ἐν V Ald.
p. 86,19 σηραγγώδεα] οὔτε σηραγγώδεα Frob.E: σηραιτώδεα V: οὐ σκληρώδεα Ho²: οὔτε σκληρώδεα Ald.N
p. 88,19 καπυρὸν] εὔπριστον Frob.E
p. 90,10 τελευτῶσά πῃ] τελευταῖον σάπη Frob.: τελευταῖον ἐσάπη E
p. 90,15 διαπριωτῷ Frob.E: διαπρίω τῷ V Ald.
p. 90,15 ἐπιλελειμμένῳ Frob.E: ἐπιλελημμένῳ V Ald.
p. 90,33 πάχιστον] παχύτατον Frob.E

In E there are a number of idiosyncratic readings, most of which are obviously the result of attempts to improve the text:

p. 66,9 αὐταὶ – 10 ἐσφλάσιος] αὗται ἐπὶ σφῶν αὐτῶν γινόμεναι ἐν τῷ ὀστέῳ τὰ νεῦρα ἀγμῆς τε καὶ φλάσιος καὶ ἔσω ἐσφλάσιος V Frob.: βλάπτουσιν ἐπὶ σφῶν αὐτῶν γινόμεναι ἐν τῷ ὀστέῳ τὰ νεῦρα. ἀγμῆς τε καὶ φλάσιος καὶ ἔσω ἐσφλάσιος δέονται E
p. 66,25 παντοῖαι] τοῖαι Frob.: τοιαῦται E
p. 70,12 αἵ – βαθύτεραι] καὶ δ' αὐταὶ καὶ βαθύτεραί V Frob.: αὐταὶ δὲ καὶ βαθύτεραί E
p. 82,14 ἄλλως – 17 ἐκκαθήρας] ἄλλως ὁρῶν δεῖ ... τὸ τίκτον ... δεύσαντα ... ὑποτείνας ... τέγξας ... καταπλάσας ... ἀπολύσας ἐκκαθήρας V: ἄλλως ὁρῶν. δεῖ ... τήκων ... δεύσας τι ... ὑποτείνας ... τέγξας ... καταπλάσας ... ἀπολύσας καὶ ἐκκαθήρας Frob.: ὅλως ὁρῶν δύνῃ. δεῖ ... τήκειν ... δεῦσαι τι ... ὑποτείνειν ... τέγξαντα ... καταπλάσαντα ... ἀπολύσαντα καὶ ἐκκαθήραντα E

g) Stemmata

Stemma for the text pp. 62,1–84,25

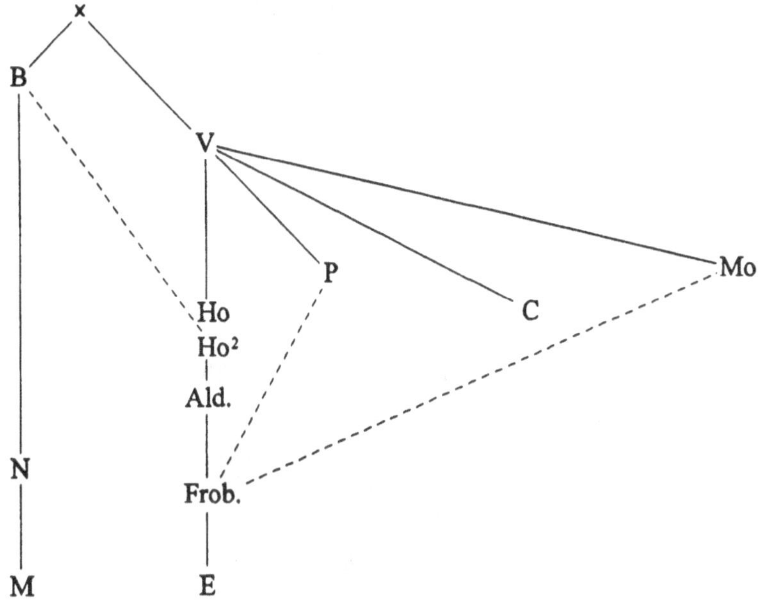

Stemma for the text pp. 84,25–92,9

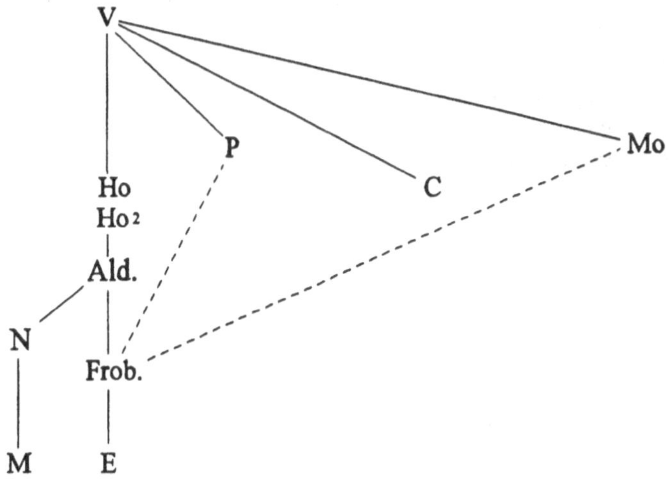

II. Indirect tradition

a) Erotian

Erotian's dictionary of Hippocratic terms has eight entries generally accepted to be from De capitis vulneribus:

B 8 (p. 28,10–14 Nachmanson): βλιχῶδες· οἱ δὲ γλισχρῶδες. Ἐπικλῆς μέν φησι τὸ λελιπασμένον μετὰ γλοιώδους ὑγρασίας ἀκαθάρτου, Εὐφορίων δὲ τὸ ἐκπεπιεσμένον καὶ κατάξηρον. Βακχεῖος δὲ καὶ Λυσίμαχος διὰ τοῦ π γράφουσι πλιχῶδες, σημᾶναι θέλοντες τὸ ἐξεπτυγμένον. (= p. 88,6)

Δ 11 (p. 33,4–6 Nachmanson): δῖνος· σκότωσις, ὡς φέρεσθαι δοκεῖν τὰ ὁρώμενα. ἔστι δὲ καὶ εἶδος ὀρχήσεως. καὶ ὁ σκοτόδινος δὲ ταὐτὸν σημαίνει καὶ ἡ σκοτοδινία. (= p. 76,9)

Δ 12 (p. 33,7 Nachmanson): διατρίβειν· ἐγχρονίζειν. (= p. 88,18)

Ε 64 (p. 40,13 Nachmanson): ἐπικαρσίην· πλαγίαν. (= p. 62,8)

Π 41 (p. 72,7–10 Nachmanson): πελλόν· ὑπόφαιον. ἀγνοοῦντες δέ τινες γράφουσι πελιόν. ὡς καὶ Σοφοκλῆς ἐν Ποιμέσι καὶ ἐν Ἀμφιαράῳ φησί· κυνὸς πελλῆς τε μηκάδος βοὸς ῥινέων. (= p. 88,7)

Π 43 (p. 72,12 Nachmanson): περκνόν· μέλαν. (= p. 88,8)

Σ 43 (p. 80,16–18 Nachmanson): συγκλέπτεται ἡ ῥαφή· ἀντὶ τοῦ παραλογίζεται, ὡς καὶ ἐν ε' Ἐπιδημιῶν φησιν· 'ἔκλεψαν δέ μου τὴν γνώμην αἱ ῥαφαὶ τοῦ βέλεος ἐν ἑαυταῖς ἔχουσαι τὸ σίνος'. = Κ 50 (p. 54,2–4 Nachmanson): κλέπτεται ἡ ῥαφή· etc. (= p. 76,14)

Υ 15 (p. 89,7 Nachmanson): ὕπομβρον ὀστέον· ὑπόνομον καὶ κάθυγρον γεγονός. (= p. 84,6)

The entry on βλιχῶδες may contain our earliest reference to De capitis vulneribus, the probable mention of this word in the glossary of the early third century lexicographer, Bacchius.

Another entry in Erotian's collection is important because it names De capitis vulneribus and quotes a passage from this text (p. 76,3–4): Ε 30 (p. 37,9–15 Nachmanson): ἕδρη· ... ἐν γοῦν τῷ Περὶ τῶν ἐν κεφαλῇ τραυμάτων αὐτὸς ἐξηγεῖται λέγων· 'διακοπὴ δὲ καὶ ἕδρη ταὐτόν ἐστιν. φλᾷ δὲ οὐ (ὅλα δ' εὖ codd.: sec. Hipp. corr. Klein) μάλα.'

b) Galen

1. Glossary

In his Glossary of Hippocratic terms, Galen gives the following entries which probably come from De capitis vulneribus[1]:

XIX 121,6–7 K.: μέλανι φαρμάκῳ· τοῦτο πῶς σκευάζεται ἐν τῷ Περὶ ἑλκῶν αὐτὸς ἐδίδαξεν. (= p. 82,15)

[1] It is unlikely that the entry XIX 94,16 K.: ἐγκάς· ἐν βάθει. refers to ἑκὰς (p. 68,16), as Foes suggests (see A. Foesius, Oeconomia Hippocratis, Frankfurt, 1588, p. 176). For the word ἐγκάς with the meaning given by Galen is not appropriate to the context of this passage. In general, the deeper a fracture extends into the bone, the larger and more obvious it is on the surface.

XIX 129,7–9 K.: πέλλα· πελία, ὑπόκιρρα. τὰ δὲ αὐτὰ καὶ πελιρὰ ὀνομάζει. Ζηνόδοτος δὲ ἐν ταῖς ἐθνικαῖς λέξεσι Σικυωνίους φησὶ τὸ κιρρόν, πέλλον ὀνομάζειν. (= p. 88,7)

XIX 140,10 K.: στεῖλαι· ἐπικαλύψαι, ἐπιχρῖσαι. (= p. 82,16)

XIX 149,9 K.: ὕπομβρον· ὕφυγρον, ὑπόπυον. (= p. 84,6)

XIX 154,8 K.: χαράκτωρι· ὠξυσμένῳ ὑπὸ τοῦ χαρακτῆρος. (= p. 90,26)

Also in the Glossary occur two entries in which reference is made to a no longer existing appendix to De capitis vulneribus (XIX 95,9–11; 144,4–7 K.; see below, p. 51). That Galen had such secondary materials at his disposal is shown also by a remark in the preface to his commentary on De diaeta acutorum (In Hipp. De victu acut. comm. IV prooem.: CMG V 9,1, p. 271,18–20).

2. In Hippocratis De officina medici comm. I 6

In Galen's Commentary on the Hippocratic treatise De officina medici (I 6: XVIII B 672,9–673,1 K.) occurs the following resumé of De capitis vulneribus's organization of head injury classification, with quotations from chapters 4–7: ... ὥσπερ κἀν τῷ Περὶ ἐν τῇ κεφαλῇ τραυμάτων αὐτὸς διῆλθε τοὺς τρόπους, καθ' οὓς αἱ πληγαὶ γίγνονται κατὰ τήνδε τὴν ῥῆσιν· «Τιτρώσκεται δὲ ὀστέον τὸ ἐν τῇ κεφαλῇ κατὰ τόσους τρόπους.» (p. 66,19) καὶ ἐφεξῆς πάλιν· «τῶν δὲ τρόπων ἑκάστου πλείονες ἰδέαι γίνονται τοῦ κατάγματος ἐν τῇ τρώσει.» (p. 66,19–20) καὶ μετὰ ταῦτα πάλιν· «Θλασθείη δ' αὐτὸ ὀστέον μόνον ἐν τῇ αὐτοῦ φύσει καὶ ῥωγμὴ τῇ θλάσει οὐκ ἂν προσγένοιτο ἐν τῷ ὀστέῳ οὐδεμία. δεύτερος οὗτος τρόπος·» (p. 68,7–8) εἶτ' ἐφεξῆς ἄλλον εἰπὼν ἐπιφέρει· «τρίτος οὗτος τρόπος·» (p. 68,22) καὶ πάλιν· «τέταρτος οὗτος τρόπος·» (p. 70,1) ἐφεξῆς· «πέμπτος οὗτος τρόπος» (p. 70,3) ἀπορώτατος φαίνεται.

3. Commentary on Hippocrates' De capitis vulneribus

In his Methodus medendi (VI 6: X 444,12–16 K.), preceding a discussion described as supplementary to the content of De capitis vulneribus, Galen announces his intention to write commentaries on Hippocratic treatises, including De capitis vulneribus. And relevant statements in the introduction to his second commentary on Epidemics III (CMG V 10,2,1, pp. 60,16–61,6) and in his bibliographical work, De libris propriis 6 (Scr. min. II 112,13–17; 113,5–7 Müller = XIX 35,3–6; 36,3–4 K.), show clearly that he had, in fact, written a commentary on De capitis vulneribus.[1]

[1] The existence of this commentary is attested by Ḥunayn ibn Isḥāq, who mentions in his missive to ʿAlī ibn Yaḥyā about the Syriac and Arabic translations of Galen's works that he has translated the work, consisting of one book, into Syriac and that also a translation by Aijūb may have existed; see Ḥunain, no. 94. Neither of these translations has survived.

This commentary has not survived. However, a quotation from it occurs in scholia which were added to the text of Oribasius by later hands in manuscripts Laurentianus Gr. 74,7 (= U; 10th c.) and Vaticanus Gr. 1885 (= R; 14th c.), Coll. med. rel. XLVI 7,1: CMG VI 2,1, p. 216,28: ὅτι διὰ τὴν ἐκ τῆς μήλης (μιλης U²) σημείωσιν εἴρηται, ὡς αὐτὸς (sc. Heliodorus) ἐν τοῖς Χειρουργουμένοις φησίν· ἀλλὰ καὶ ὁ Γαληνὸς ἐν τῷ (το U²) ὑπο(μνήματι) τοῦ Περὶ σημείων (σιμιων U²) τῶν ἐν κεφαλῇ τρωμάτων φησίν· μήλωσιν δὲ ὀνομάζει τὴν διὰ τῆς μηλωτίδος ἐπίσκεψιν ἣν ποιούμεθα καθέντες αὐτὴν ἔσω U²;[1] ἀντὶ τῇ σημειώσει· φησὶ γὰρ ὁ Γαληνὸς ἐν τῷ τοῦ (del. Raeder) Περὶ τῶν ἐν κεφαλῇ τρωμάτων· μήλωσιν δ' ὀνομάζει τὴν διὰ τῆς μηλωτίδος ἐπίσκεψιν ἣν ποιούμεθα καθέντες αὐτὴν ἔσω R²

Oribasius himself may have preserved other parts of the commentary. From his text, presented under the heading Ἐκ τῶν Γαληνοῦ. Περὶ τῶν ἐν κεφαλῇ καταγμάτων (Coll. med. rel. XLVI 21: CMG VI 2,1, p. 227,25–232,17) only a few passages can be proven to be excerpts from writings of Galen that have survived: p. 228,31–229,20 = Meth. med. VI 6: X 445,7–446,17 K.; p. 229,24–230,1 = 448,4–17; 449,6–7 K.; p. 230,13–31 = 449,18–450,2. 10–14; 451,15–452,8; 454,1 K.; p. 231,12–14 = 454,2–5 K.; p. 231,14–19 = De simpl. med. temp. et fac. X 2: XII 255,9–15; 256,14–257,1 K.; p. 231,19–24 = Meth. med. VI 6: X 454,5–10; 455,9–12 K. For the remaining passages (pp. 227,25–228,31; 229,20–24; 230,1–13. 31–231,12. 24–232,17) the possibility must be considered that they were taken from the commentary on De capitis vulneribus. On the basis of content there are two general sections, one on classification of skull injuries and one on treatment. The section on classification contains reference to a phrase in De capitis vulneribus: ἕδραν γὰρ καὶ διακοπὴν ταὐτὸν εἶναί φησιν Ἱπποκράτης (p. 227,27), which appears three times in the Hippocratic text (pp. 72,5; 76,3–4; 78,3–4). And in both sections there are echoes of statements from the Hippocratic treatise which suggest that the passages do originate in the lost commentary of Galen, e.g. CMG VI 2,1, p. 228, 27–28 ἐξ ἀνάγκης σύνεστι τῇ ῥωγμῇ καὶ θλάσις, cf. p. 66,21–22 τῇ ῥωγμῇ ... ἀνάγκη φλάσιν προσγενέσθαι; p. 228,28–29 ἕδρα μέντοι καὶ θλάσις ἅμα δύναται γίνεσθαι χωρὶς ῥωγμῆς, cf. p. 70,2 ῥωγμὴ δὲ οὐκ ἂν προσγένοιτο τῇ ἕδρῃ καὶ τῇ φλάσει; p. 231,10–11 δεῖ δὲ μηδέποτε τὴν τρίτην ἀπὸ τῆς ἀρχῆς ἡμέραν ὑπερβῆναι, ἀλλ' εἶναι τοῦτον ὅρον ἐξωτάτω, cf. p. 82, 5–7 ἣν μὲν δοκῇ ἐς πρῖσιν ἀφήκειν ἡ τρῶσις τοῦ ὀστέου, πρίειν χρὴ καὶ τὰς τρεῖς ἡμέρας μὴ ὑπερβάλλειν ἀπρίωτον; p. 231,26–27 τὰ χωρὶς ἀνατρήσεως δ' ἕλκη καὶ αὐτά, καθ' ὅσον οἷόν τε πειρᾶσθαι χρὴ θεραπεύειν ἄνευ ἐπιδέσμων, cf. p. 78,15 οὐδ' ἐπιδεῖν χρὴ ἕλκος ἐν κεφαλῇ.

This thesis is supported by scholia entered next to these passages by R². These scholia offer, under the title Περὶ τῶν ἐν τῇ κεφαλῇ τρωμάτων, word for word quotations from the Hippocratic text, with only minor deviations. These quotations are, with one exception, marked by the introductory ῥητοῦ ("from the lemma") as quotations from the lemmas of a commentary. That the commentary is that of Galen is clear from the fact, that, even though no au-

1 The deviations from the wording provided by Raeder are based on a recent reading of the text of the scholion in U by J. Kollesch and D. Nickel.

thor of the quotations is named, they are part of a section for which as a whole Galen is the stated source.

The scholia read as follows:

p. 227,25 ἀπὸ τοῦ Περὶ τῶν ἐν τῇ κεφαλῇ τρωμάτων, ῥητοῦ· αἱ δ' ἕδραι τῶν ὀξέων (p. 66,9)

p. 228,22 ἀπὸ τοῦ αὐτοῦ, ῥητοῦ· ὀστέον τιτρώσκεται ἄλλῃ τῆς κεφαλῆς (p. 70,18)

p. 228,26 ἀπὸ τοῦ αὐτοῦ, ῥητοῦ· καὶ ἕδρη τοῦ βέλεος γίνεται ἐν τῷ ὀστέῳ (p. 70,3–4)

p. 229,20 ἀπὸ τοῦ ⟨Περὶ τῶν⟩ ἐν τῇ κεφαλῇ τρωμάτων, ῥητοῦ· τουτέων τὸν τρόπον τῆς κατήξιος (p. 70,23)

p. 230,8 ἀπὸ τοῦ αὐτοῦ· ἀλλ' οὐ χρὴ τὰς ῥαφὰς αὐτὰς πρίειν (p. 78,10)

p. 230,31 ἀπὸ τοῦ Περὶ τῶν ἐν τῇ κεφαλῇ τρωμάτων, ῥητοῦ· ἔπειτα διαμοτῶσαι πᾶν τὸ ἕλκος (p. 80,19)

p. 231,3 ἀπὸ τοῦ αὐτοῦ Περὶ τῶν ἐν τῇ κεφαλῇ τρωμάτων, ῥητοῦ· ἄλλως τε καὶ τῆς θερμῆς ὥρης (p. 82,7)

p. 231,5 ἀπὸ τοῦ αὐτοῦ, ῥητοῦ· ἔπειτα διαμοτῶσαι πᾶν τὸ ἕλκος (p. 80,19)

p. 231,24 ἀπὸ τοῦ αὐτοῦ, Περὶ τῶν ἐν τῇ κεφαλῇ τρωμάτων, ῥητοῦ· οὐδὲ ἐπιδεῖν χρὴ ἕλκος ἐν κεφαλῇ (p. 78,15)

p. 232,1 ἀπὸ τοῦ αὐτοῦ, ῥητοῦ· ἢν μὴ ἐν τῷ μετώπῳ ᾖ τὸ ἕλκος (p. 78,16)[1]

On the basis of a similar scholiast's note another passage in Oribasius (Coll. med. rel. XLIII 38,3: CMG VI 2,1, p. 102,1–5) may be assigned to Galen's commentary:

p. 102,1 ἀπὸ τοῦ Περὶ τῶν ἐν κεφαλῇ τραυμάτων, ῥητοῦ· καὶ τὰ κυκλοτερέα τῶν ἑλκῶν (p. 80,6)

The quotations of the lemmas suggest that Galen's commentary was still available to the scholiast to the same extent as it had been to Oribasius.

III. Editions and translations

a) The Aldine edition

The first printed edition in Greek of the collected Hippocratic works, titled Omnia opera Hippocratis, was published by the Aldine press in Venice in 1526 (= Ald.). Its editor was Franciscus Asulanus. **Ald.**

The treatise De capitis vulneribus is located on fol. 191^{v}–194^{r} and 196^{r}. The sections of De aere aquis locis, which are found with De capitis vulneri-

[1] The quotations reflect the tradition of B: p. 78,15 ἐπιδειν B schol.: πιέζειν V; p. 80,19 παν το ελκος B schol.: τὸ ἕλκος πᾶν V.

bus in the manuscript V, are here separated from the body of De capitis vulneribus by the title, Ταῦτα προσγεγράφθαι τῷδε τῷ βιβλίῳ, Γαληνός φησι. This section concludes with the words, πρὸς τὸν γινόμενον ὀρρόν (p. 92,1–2). The following last lines of De capitis vulneribus (p. 92,3 Καὶ – 8 γέγραπται) are separated from the sections of De aere aquis locis by the title, Καὶ τάδε τὰ τελευταῖα ὑπό τινος προσγεγράφθαι δῆλον ἐστίν.

For the edition of De capitis vulneribus Asulanus used as his model the manuscript Ho as revised for printing by Ho^2. This is clearly shown by the readings which are peculiar to the Aldine edition and to Ho / Ho^2, the only testimony to these readings that predates the Aldine.

1. Omissions

p. 64,3	τοῦ^{II} om. Ho Ald.
p. 66,12	ὁ om. Ho Ald.
p. 68,8	τρόπος om. Ho Ald.
p. 68,10	διὰ – 11 τε καὶ^{I} om. Ho Ald.
p. 68,16	τε om. Ho Ald.
p. 76,3	τὸ om. Ho Ald.
p. 78,8	ὁ om. Ho Ald.
p. 80,22	δὲ^{II} del. Ho^2, om. Ald.
p. 82,22	μέλαιναν del. Ho^2, om. Ald.
p. 84,10	καὶ^{II} – σφυγμὸν om. Ho Ald.
p. 84,11	κακὰ om. Ho Ald.
p. 84,22	ὑγρὴ om. Ho Ald.
p. 92,9	ἣν – πρίεις del. Ho^2, om. Ald.

2. Addition

p. 82,17	post ἀπολύσας add. καὶ Ho^2 Ald.

3. Wrong readings

p. 64,22	ὑπὸ λεπτοτάτῳ] ὑπολεπτοτάτω Ho^2 Ald.
p. 64,28	τὸ^{I} – ὄπισθεν] τοῦ ὀστέου παντὸς τὸ ὀστέον Ho^2 Ald.
p. 70,15	μένῃ] μένει Ho Ald.
p. 78,27	τι σίνος] τὸ σίνος Ho Ald.
p. 80,22	μάζῃ] μάζην Ho Ald.

4. Corrections or attempted corrections

p. 64,7	σκληρότητος ... μαλθακότητος ... κοιλότητος] σκληρότητι ... μαλθακότητι ... κοιλότητι Ho^2 Ald.
p. 80,22	δὲ μάσσειν] διαμάσσειν Ho^2 Ald.
p. 82,15	τὸ τηκτὸν] τήκων Ho^2 Ald.
p. 82,15	δεύσαντα] δεύσας τι Ho^2 Ald.
p. 86,13	διάπυον] διαπύον Ho^2 Ald.
p. 86,14	ποιήσειεν] ποιήσηται Ho^2 Ald.
p. 86,19	σηραγγώδεα] οὐ σκληρώδεα Ho^2: οὔτε σκληρώδεα Ald.
p. 88,9	ἅπαν ὠχρὸν] ἔπωχρον Ho^2 Ald.
p. 88,10	ἐπιλαμβάνει Ho Ald.

Readings of B, occasionally found in the text of the Aldine, also go back to the collations of that manuscript undertaken by Ho² for the printing, e.g.:

p. 74,16 ἀντίον B Ho² Ald.: ἐναντίον V Ho
p. 78,10 ἀποχωρήσαντα B Ho² Ald.: ἀποχωρίσαι τὰ V Ho
p. 78,14 τέγγειν B Ho² Ald.: τείνειν V Ho
p. 80,16 εἴ τι ἔχει B Ho² Ald.: ἐπέχει V Ho
p. 84,6 ὑπόπυον B Ho² Ald.: ὑπὸ πύϑη V Ho

The agreement between the text of the Aldine and that of its manuscript model extends even to peculiarities of orthography and the use of the breathings, e.g.: p. 64,15 ῥίγνυται Ho Ald.; p. 68,24 ἐπιπαλαιότερον Ho Ald.; p. 80, 20 εὐρύτατον Ho Ald.

Of the few differences between the Aldine text and that of Ho several can be explained as printing errors, e.g.: p. 62,18 τελευτῶσα Ho: τελευτῶσαι Ald.; p. 80,3–4 καὶ ὅταν τὸ μὲν] κακὸν ἂν μὲν τὸ μὲν Ho: κακὸν et μὲν^{I} punctis del. et καὶ in marg. add. Ho²: ἂν καὶ τὸ μὲν Ald.[1]; p. 80,15–16 ὀστέου ... ἐψιλωμένου] ὀστέον ... ἐψιλωμένον Ald.; p. 88,8 τηνικαῦτα Ho: τηνικαῦται Ald.; p. 90,16 λειπόμενον Ho: λοιπόμενον Ald.; p. 90,32 ὅπη Ho: ὅτη Ald.; p. 90,33 πάχιστον] πάχυστον Ald.; p. 92,4 τὴν Ho: καὶ Ald. The remaining differences probably represent changes made by the editor during printing and not indicated on the manuscript: p. 62,18 τῇσι μακρῇσι γραμμῇσι Ho: τὴν μακρὴν γραμμήν Ald.; p. 70,25 γενομένης Ald.: γενομένη Ho; p. 74,6 ἀσϑενέστερον] ἀσϑενεστέρως Ho: ἀσϑενεστέρους Ald.; p. 80,17 τομήν] τολίην Ho: ὠτείλην Ald.; p. 82,12 καὶ^{III} add. Ald.; p. 88,13 τὰ] τὸ Ho: τὰ Ald.

b) The Froben edition

The first Froben edition of Hippocrates, titled, Hippocratis Coi ... libri omnes ..., was published in Basle in 1538 (= Frob.). Its editor was Janus Cornarius who announces in his Preface that he used the Aldine as the basic text for his complete edition of the Hippocratic writings and in addition for corrections referred to three manuscripts. With more or less probability these can be identified as Palatinus Gr. 192 (= P), Monacensis Gr. 71 (= Mo) and Parisinus Gr. 2255 (= E).[2] **Frob.**

The treatise De capitis vulneribus is contained on pp. 445–451 and 456. The arrangement concerning the insertion of the passages of De aere aquis locis (p. 92,1) is identical to that of the Aldine edition (see above, pp. 39–40).

In the text of the Froben edition most of those readings occur which were encountered for the first time in the Aldine, including several printing

1 The editor's intent was surely that καὶ replace κακὸν, not μὲν.

2 See above, pp. 26–28; 28 n. 4; Rivier, p. 154 n. 6. At the time Cornarius may have used E, this manuscript almost certainly did not contain De cap. vuln. (see above, pp. 33–34). There can be no doubt that Cornarius made use of manuscripts. In the copy of the 1526 Aldine edition of Hippocrates, now in the University Library of Göttingen (see below, p. 46 n. 1), there are notes, marginal emendations and subtitles identical to those of Mo, all in the hand of Cornarius (see Rivier, pp. 176–177).

errors: p. 62,18 τελευτῶσα] τελευτῶσαι Ald. Frob.; τῇσι μακρῇσι γραμμῇσιν] τὴν μακρὴν γραμμήν Ald. Frob.; p. 74,6 ἀσθενέστερον] ἀσθενεστέρους Ald. Frob.; p. 80,3 καὶ ὅταν] ἂν καὶ Ald. Frob.; p. 80,17 τομήν] ὠτείλην Ald. Frob.; p. 88,13 τὰ Ald. Frob.; p. 92,4 τὴν] καὶ Ald. Frob.

Differences from the text of the Aldine are in part corrections which were made with the use of manuscripts, and in part independent emendations of the editor. The two passages missing in the Aldine text and supplied in the Froben are certainly based on manuscript authority: p. 68,10 διὰ – 11 τε καὶ[I] om. Ald.: διὰ παντὸς τοῦ ὀστέου, καὶ ἧσσον ἐς βαθὺ, καὶ διὰ παντὸς τοῦ ὀστέου, καὶ ἐπὶ πλέον τε καὶ add. Frob.; p. 84,10 καὶ[II] – σφυγμὸν om. Ald., add. Frob. In the first case the wording concurs with that of the V-tradition, in which the οὐ before διὰ παντὸς in B is missing, and so makes it likely that the manuscript P or Mo served as the source for the passage. Also, the correction p. 90,15 διαπριωτῷ in place of διαπρίω τῷ, found first in P and otherwise only in the Froben, further supports the use of P.

The following readings, since they do not occur elsewhere in the tradition, must undoubtedly be considered independent textual emendations of Cornarius: p. 64,9 post λεπτότητι add. οὕτως Frob.; p. 66,25 παντοῖαι] τοῖαι Frob.; p. 70,19 ἕβδομος] πέμπτος Frob.; p. 80,15–16 τοῦ ὀστέου ... ἐψιλωμένου] ὀστέον ... ἐψιλωμένον Ald.: ὀστέων ... ἐψιλωμένων Frob.; p. 82,20 μέλαν ἐόν Frob.: μελάνεον B V Ald.; p. 84,30 ἀποστρακωθὲν] ἀπεστρακὸς, ἐν V Ald.: ἀποστρακὸς, ἐν Frob.; p. 86,19 σηραγγώδεα] σηραιτώδεα V: οὔτε σκληρώδεα Ald.: οὔτε σηραγγώδεα Frob.; p. 88,19 καπυρὸν] εὔπριστον Frob.; p. 90,10 τελευτῶσά πῃ] τελευταῖον σάπῃ Frob.; p. 90,15 ἐπιλελειμμένῳ Frob.: ἐπιλελημμένῳ V Ald.; p. 90,33 πάχιστον] πάχυστον Ald.: παχύτατον Frob.

The following readings may also possibly be those of the editor. Although they correspond to the readings in B, they are of a sort that could be conjectured from context without manuscript authority by an expert like Cornarius: p. 64,2 σηραγγῶδες Frob.: σειραιτῶδες V Ald.; p. 64,18 ἀποθνήσκει[1] Frob.: ἀποθνήσκειν V Ald.; p. 70,23 φλάσις Frob.: φάσις V Ald.; p. 72,17 ἔργου Frob.: ἐρίου V Ald.; p. 80,28 αὖτις] αὖθις Frob.; p. 82,3 προσγένηται Frob.: προστένηται V Ald.

c) Editions published after the Froben

Only those editions are listed which are of importance with regard to the text or at least reveal the editors' interest in textual problems[2]:

Hippocratis ... De capitis vulneribus liber, Latinitate donatus a F. Vertuniano (F. de Saint-Vertunien) ... Ejusdem Hippocratis textus Graecus a J. Scaligero castigatus, cum ipsius Scaligeri castigationum suarum explicatione, Paris, 1578

Joseph Juste Scaliger was in the early years of his career as a textual

[1] The same correction is found in C and Ho2.

[2] Petrequin, pp. 432–433, provides a list of the older editions, translations and commentaries.

critic. His emendations, often insensitive to the medical context, are too many and too rash. But later commentators frequently respond to his emendations and therefore they must be recounted.

Hippocratis Coi Opera ... Graece et Latine a H. Mercuriali ... restituta, Venice, 1588, vol. I, pp. 245–259

This edition repeats in essence the Froben text and the translation of Cornarius (see below, pp. 45–46). The variants, provided in the margins and designated "Vet. Cod.", offer nothing beyond the known manuscript sources and the emendations of Scaliger.

Magni Hippocratis ... Opera omnia quae extant ... Latina interpretatione et annotationibus illustrata A. Foesio ... authore ... His praeterea accessere variae ... lectiones Graecae ..., Frankfurt, 1595, sectio VI, pp. 172–192

The text of this edition is very close to that of the Froben. In his notes Foes discusses divergent readings and on col. 224 offers variants which had become known to him as handwritten entries in copies of the Aldine and Froben editions owned by A. Févré and L. Servin. These variants are unproductive for textual reconstruction. On cols. 248–251 variants are listed which according to Foes stem in large part from a Codex Mediceus, preserved in Paris in the library of Catherine de' Medici (see cols. 225/226); this manuscript is probably to be identified as N. Foes' edition also contains noteworthy comments and emendations by J. Martin, professor of medicine in Paris (cols. 252–253) and Aemilius Portus, Heidelberg scholar (in an unpaginated supplement, titled "Variae Lectiones"). The Latin translation was published separately later under the title, Magni Hippocratis ... Opera omnia quae extant ... Latina interpretatione donata, ac denuo separatim in lucem edita A. Foesio ... authore ..., Frankfurt, 1596, pp. 916–929.

Hippocratis Coi Chirurgia ... Graece restituta et commentariis illustrata ..., ed. E. Maniaud, Paris, 1619, pp. 290–427

The commentary on De capitis vulneribus contains discussions of textual difficulties with references to manuscript readings and to suggestions of Scaliger and Foesius.

Hippocratis Coi sive magni Opera omnia Graece et Latine, ed. J. A. van der Linden, Leiden, 1665, vol. II, pp. 687–708

Œuvres complètes d'Hippocrate, ed. and transl. E. Littré, vol. III, Paris, 1841, pp. 182–261

As the first edition to deal systematically and consistently with textual problems, this edition represents an important advance over its predecessors. Its drawbacks lie in the fact that, for the text of De capitis vulneribus, Littré relied exclusively on the Parisian manuscripts and that he gave undue prominence to the textual comments in Foes' edition, including the variants of Févré and Servin. The manuscript designated B by Littré is the Codex Mediceus utilized by Foes (cf. above); the readings from it quoted by Littré correspond to those in the statements of Foes. This source, B, therefore is not identical to Laurentianus 74,7 (= B).

Hippocratis et aliorum medicorum veterum reliquiae, ed. F. Z. Ermerins, vol. I, Utrecht, 1859, pp. 367–394

This edition is based on that of Littré. Ermerins makes many emendations, some of which warrant serious consideration.

Ἱπποκράτης κομιδῇ, ed. K. H. Th. Reinhold, vol. I, Athens, 1865, pp. 37–56

Reinhold's text is interesting because of its vigorous emendations of difficult passages. However, these emendations are often so drastic as to be rewritings, taking too little account of the manuscript readings.

J. E. Petrequin, Chirurgie d'Hippocrate, vol. I, Paris, 1877, pp. 434–523

This edition contains, apart from the Greek text, a French translation and copious notes. In general the text follows that of Littré; however, Petrequin has an extreme reluctance to alter the transmitted text. As a result he rejects some good emendations and defends some clearly corrupt passages. But his discussions of textual problems are thorough and he includes his correspondence with Littré on some of these passages.

Hippocratis Opera quae feruntur omnia, ed. H. Kühlewein, vol. II, Leipzig, 1902, pp. 1–29

This edition is distinguished by its careful and thorough use of the earliest manuscripts, B and V, which served here for the first time as main sources for the text.

Hippocrates with an English translation, vol. III, ed. E. T. Withington, London and Cambridge, Mass., 1928 (Loeb Classical Library), pp. 6–51

This translation is sensitive to the textual problems.

d) The Latin translations

From the 16th c. come the following Latin translations of De capitis vulneribus, published either together with the Greek text or separately:

Hippocratis Coi ... octoginta volumina ... per M. Fabium Calvum ... latinitate donata ..., Rome, 1525, pp. 663–676 (this translation was used in the edition: Hippocratis Coi ... Opera per Fabium Calvum, Guil. Copum, Nicolaum Leonicenum et Andream Brentium latinitate donata, Basle, 1526, pp. 449–454)

The translation of De capitis vulneribus is rough and, at times, inaccurate. It follows the text of V: p. 68,14 ἢ μὴ πέφλασται om. V Calv.; p. 70,1 καὶ – 3 τρόπος om. V Calv.; p. 72,7 εἴτ' – ἰσχυροτέροισιν om. V Calv.; p. 76,26 οὔτε – 27 διαχαλάσῃ om. V Calv. The large fragments of De aere aquis locis incorporated in V at p. 92,1 are translated by Calvus in the same location with no distinguishing break or title. The translation of Calvus is preceded by a brief introductory section, found in none of the nine extant manuscripts (see below, pp. 94–95, the note to p. 62,3). Although the source of these sentences remains unknown, there is nothing in the rest of the translation to suggest use of another Greek manuscript, now lost.

Chirurgia e Graeco in Latinum conversa, V. Vidio (G. Guidi) Florentino interprete, cum nonnullis eiusdem Vidii commentariis, Paris, 1544, pp. 61–126 (the translation of De capitis vulneribus was later published separately: Hippocrates, De vulneribus capitis, Paris, 1550)

A handwritten predecessor of this translation of De capitis vulneribus and of the commentary on it is found in codex Parisinus Lat. 6861. It was copied by Christophe Auer in Rome, probably in 1541/1542, before Guidi went to Paris (cf. above, p. 25) and bears the title, Hippocrates de vulneribus capitis a Vido Vidio Florentino in Latinum versus et emendatus. It must be regarded as a specimen by which Guidi wished to demonstrate to his royal benefactor, Francis I, his progress on the collected surgical works.

Translation and commentary are essentially identical in the handwritten and printed versions. The differences in the translation consist of minor changes in word order, occasional substitution of synonyms, and, in rare cases, the reformulation of a phrase.

The Froben edition appears to have served as the basis for the translation. This can be deduced from passages where the Latin version offers equivalents for variant readings which (apart from the manuscript E which is also derived from the Froben) are found exclusively in the Froben text: p. 70, 19 ἕβδομος V Ald.: εβδομαιος B: πέμπτος Frob.: quintus Guidi; p. 88,19 καπυρὸν V Ald.: εὔπριστον Frob.: facile … secatur Guidi; p. 90,10 τελευτῶσά πη V Ald.: τελευταῖον σάπη Frob.: tandem putresceret Guidi.

Guidi states in his note to the reader, prefacing this 1544 edition, that, for passages he considered faulty, he used the most ancient manuscripts, especially those in the collection of his patron, Cardinal Ridolfi. This is corroborated by his translation; where the Froben has corrupt passages of the V-traditon (either omissions or wrong readings) Guidi has supplied corrections from the B-tradition: p. 66,10 ἄνευ ῥωγμῆς BNM: neque findatur Guidi: τὰ νεῦρα ἀγμῆς V Ald. Frob.; p. 70,1–3 και εδρη μεν αν γενοιτο φλασιν εχουσα του ὀστεου περι αὐτην ρωγμη δε οὐκ προσγενοιτο τη εδρη και τη φλασει ὑπο του βελεος· πεμπτος οὑτος τροπος BNM: Potest et collidi os quod inciditur, quamvis nulla colliso incisoque rima superveniat Guidi: om. V Ald. Frob.; p. 76,26–27 ουτε ην φλασθεντος του ὀστεου κατα τας σαρκας ραγη και διαχαλασθη BNM: neque ubi sutura finditur et resolvitur, propterea quod os et caro collidatur Guidi: om. V Ald. Frob. In Rome Guidi certainly had access to B, a manuscript known to him (see above, p. 14 n. 6), probably to N and possibly to M if that manuscript was complete at the time. That he may have used N or M in lieu of B or, for the last part of the treatise missing in B, may have used either N or M or the Aldine edition is suggested by the following reading: p. 86,19 σηραγγώδεα] σηραιτώδεα V: οὔτε σκλήρωδεα Ald. NM: non dura Guidi: οὔτε σηραγγώδεα Frob.: deest B.

Hippocratis Coi … Opera quae extant omnia Iano Cornario interprete, Venice, 1545 (the translation was frequently reprinted; I have used the edition: Hippocratis Coi … Opera quae ad nos extant omnia per Ianum Cornarium … Latina lingua conscripta, Basle, 1546, pp. 590–597)

The text of his Greek edition of 1538 served as the basis for his translation. Also taken into account were emendations Cornarius made in his copy of the Aldine edition[1]: e.g. p. 70,23 ante Τούτων addiderit ἐκ Corn.: ex his Corn.Lat.; ἥ τε ... ἡ] ἤντε ... ἣ Corn.: tum si ... est Corn.Lat.; p. 72,23 τούτων] τούτω Ald.: τοιοῦτον Corn.: tale Corn.Lat.; p. 76,17 αὐτὴ] αὐτῇ Ald.: αὕτη Corn.: haec Corn.Lat.; p. 76,22 τὰ δ' ἄλλα] τ' ἄλλα Ald.: τὰ γὰρ ἄλλα Corn.: nam reliqua Corn.Lat.; p. 76,25 ἀπὸ ἕδρης ... γενομένης] ὑπὸ ἕδρης ... γενομένης Ald.: ὑπὸ ἕδρης ... γενομένη (sc. ῥῆξις) Corn.: si a ... sede fiat (sc. ruptio) Corn.Lat.; p. 86,9 εἰκὸς] εἶδος Corn.: forma Corn.Lat.; p. 88,8 (περκνόν,) λεῖον ἐόν] (περκνὸν) λεῖον ὂν Ald.: λίαν Corn.: valde (nigrum) Corn.Lat.; p. 90,10 τελευτῶσά πῃ καὶ διεμύδησεν] τελευταῖον ὅταν (postea supra lin. add.) σάπη no(s) h(abemus). vel lege τελευταῖον ὅταν σαπῇ γε κίνδυνος καὶ μυδήσειν Corn.: postremum ubi madore corrumpi ac putrescere ipsam periculum est Corn.Lat.

Among the entries Cornarius made in the Aldine copy is a passage in Greek which precedes the printed text and, in its content, corresponds to the introduction Calvus attached to his translation (see above, p. 44). This passage, in a Latin version, was also incorporated into Cornarius' translation (see below, pp. 94–95, the note to p. 62,3).

e) Modern translations

The medical importance of the treatise De capitis vulneribus is indicated by the fact that it was translated into modern languages (French, Italian, English, German, Dutch) as early as the mid-sixteenth century. Among the more recent translations, published without the Greek text, these are noteworthy:

The genuine works of Hippocrates, transl. F. Adams, London, 1849, vol. I, pp. 445–466 (repr. New York, 1886)

Hippokrates, Sämmtliche Werke, transl. R. Fuchs, vol. III, Munich, 1900, pp. 258–280

Opere di Ippocrate, transl. M. Vegetti, Turin, 1965, pp. 351–369

B. Dialectal characteristics in B and V

I. Phonetics

1. η for α

η in place of ᾱ is standard throughout B and V, with a few exceptions: p. 78, 15 ιησιν B: ἴασιν V; p. 82,25 πρῆγμα V: τα πραγματα B; p. 90,18 θερμασίας V (B deest). η in place of ᾰ[2] wrongly occurs at p. 62,17 βραχεῖα] βραχειη

[1] This copy is the property of the Niedersächsische Staats- und Universitätsbibliothek Göttingen. Copies of the folia containing the text of De capitis vulneribus were graciously placed at the disposal of Corpus Medicorum Graecorum.

[2] Concerning nouns it is uncertain if Ionic η has replaced original ᾱ (cf. E. Schwyzer, in: Hippokrates, Über Entstehung und Aufbau des menschlichen Körpers, p. 73 with n. 1).

(-είη) B V; p. 72,4 εὐρεῖα] ευρειη B: εὐρέη V; in these cases, the forms in η are hyperionisms. The forms in ᾰ have been accepted also at p. 62,23. 24 ὁμοιχροια B: ὁμοχροίη V; p. 76,20 ἀσθένειαν V: ασθενειην B; p. 80,9 ἀσφαλειαν B: ἀσφαλείην V.

2. Contraction

In α-contract and o-contract verbs the normal Attic-Ionic contracted forms are found in both B and V, with a few exceptions, some of which are hyperionisms: p. 72,16 ὁρῶντα V: ὁρεωντα B[1]; p. 72,22 πειρῆσθαι BV; p. 86,26 πειρῆσθαι V (deest B).

In ε-contract verbs forms with ε + ο, οι or ω are uncontracted in B and V, with three exceptions where only the text of V is extant: p. 88,17 ἐννοίης (wrongly for ἐννοοίης); p. 90,27 ἐξαιρεῦντα; p. 90,34 σκοπούμενος (here corrected to -εόμενος). Once ε + ου is wrongly contracted to ου in V: p. 90,10 κακοπαθοῦσαν.

Forms with ε + ε are sometimes contracted in both B and V. In most cases, however, in both B and V these forms as well as those with ε + η are uncontracted: p. 86,9 ἀφαιρέειν; p. 90,11 ἀφαιρέης; pp. 90,23; 92,6 ἀφελέειν; p. 92,7 ἀφικνέεσθαι; pp. 78,13; 90,33 δοκέει; pp. 78,27; 80,17. 27; 82,5 (δοκείη V); 88, 21; 90,17; 92,1 δοκέη(ι); pp. 76,3; 84,10 ἐμποιέει; p. 90,18. 23 ἐξαιρέειν; p. 82, 22 ἐπιξέειν; p. 70,4 καλέεται; p. 90,13 κινέεται; pp. 74,26; 90,21 ποιέει; p. 80, 8. 23 ποιέειν; pp. 72,16. 19; 76,7; 78,11. 15; 86,34 ποιέεσθαι; p. 74,4 περικρατέη. They have been contracted in this edition.

In σ-stem nouns and adjectives forms in ε + ο, α and ω remain open (βέλεος, ἕλκεος; βέλεα, ἕλκεα; βελέων, ἑλκέων; ἀφανέος; περιφερέα, προμήκεα, ἀφανέα; ἀφανέων) with one exception, p. 86,33 ὑγιᾶ.

Two adjective forms in ε + ε are open in both B and V, pp. 66,26; 82,1 καταφανέες; p. 78,2 ῥωγμοειδέες, and as hyperionisms have been contracted to -εῖς.[2]

The contracted pronominal form σφῶν at p. 66,9 has been changed to the Ionic σφέων.

The first declension nouns generally preserve in the genitive plural the open form after consonants in both manuscripts, e.g. pp. 66,25. 27; 68,2. 16 ῥωγμέων; p. 88,3. 15 ἡμερέων.[3] In one instance a contracted gen. pl. appears in both B and V, p. 66,18 ῥαφῶν, which has been corrected to -έων. Similar false contractions occur at p. 84,9 περιεχουσῶν B V and p. 66,10 αὐτῶν V.

The findings in De capitis vulneribus permit no clear conclusion since in both B and V forms in ᾰ as well as η have been transmitted.

1 Possible evidence for the occurrence of the stem ὁρε- is found at p. 82,14: ὁρεων B: ὁρῶν V, provided it does not arise from analogy to the false form ὁρεωντα. Unequivocal examples of both stems are found in the manuscripts of other Hippocratic texts: e.g. De nat. hom.: CMG I 1,3, p. 178,11 ὁρῶντες A: ὁρέοντες M V; p. 220,7 ἐσορῶντι A ϑ M^{m}: ἐσορέοντι M V; and the ὁρε- forms are well attested in Ionic prose (cf. Jouanna, in: CMG I 1,3, p. 140).

2 Cf. Jouanna, in: CMG I 1,3, p. 141.

3 The form σαρκέων (p. 84,9) transmitted in V is based on a phonologically unacceptable analogy.

3. Variations in phonologic phenomena

αἰεί / ἀεί:

B has αἰεί twice (p. 62,10. 13) and ἀεί once (p. 64,1); V has αἰεί twice (pp. 62, 10; 90,33) and ἀεί twice (pp. 62,13; 92,5). αἰεί is used in this edition.

αὖτις / αὖθις:

In both instances, pp. 80,28; 82,21, B has αὖθις and V αὖτις. The Ionic αὖτις is printed in this edition.

γιν- / γιγν-:

Concerning γί(γ)νεσθαι with its compounds (δια-, προσ-), B and V, where they concur, for the most part have forms in γιν-. The stem γιγν- appears once in both B and V, p. 84,17, twenty times in B, pp. 64,6. 26; 66,14. 20. 22 (προσγενέσθαι V). 25. 26; 68,9. 15. 26 (προσγενέσθαι V); 70,6. 14; 72,3 (γενομένη V); 74,3. 28; 76,11; 82,25 (γένοιτο V); 84,8. 16 (γενομένας V). 23. With (δια)γι(γ)νώσκειν there is agreement in both B and V for either stem in three instances (pp. 72,22; 80,26 διαγινώσκειν; p. 72,28 γιγνώσκειν) and difference once (p. 82,13 διαγιγνωσκης B: διαγινώσκης V). In the present edition the Ionic stem γιν- has been used throughout.

ει / ε:

εἵνεκα / ἕνεκα: Whereas V has in all cases the Ionic εἵνεκα, B has once, at p. 80,29, the Attic ἕνεκα.

ἔσω / εἴσω: Both B and V have ἔσω once, p. 72,9, and εἴσω twice, pp. 74,20; 80,30. Otherwise all examples in B (with exception of p. 74,1 εω) are εἴσω: pp. 64,15. 33 (om. V); 66,10; 68,18. 19 (om. V). 20 (εἰσσω); 70,16. 27; 72,27; 74,9. 24; 76,5, and all in V are ἔσω (including those in the later chapters, not extant in B: p. 86,4. 15. 17). However, the preposition and the prefix are, without exception, ἐς in both B and V, and therefore ἔσω has been used in this edition.[1]

μέζων / μείζων: B has only the Ionic form, μέζων, accepted for this text, while V has only the Attic, μείζων (pp. 64,31; 78,8; 84,29; 90,21).

πλείων / πλέων: As a rule, B has πλει- and V πλε-. In three instances B and V both have πλε-: pp. 66,4; 68,11; 74,29, while V only once, in agreement with B, has πλει-, in the contracted form of the fem. nom. pl. πλείους, p. 68,9. In this edition the forms given in B have been used, with the exception of ἐπὶ πλέον at p. 68,22–23 (cf. ἐπὶ πλέον at p. 68,11).[2]

ἰθύς / εὐθύς:

V has in all four cases the Ionic form, B in three cases the Attic (pp. 68,4bis; 70,10).

1 Cf. Kühlewein, vol. I, pp. CVIII–CIX; Jouanna, in: CMG I 1,3, pp. 138–139.

2 Cf. Jouanna, in: CMG I 1,3, p. 139.

ου / ο:

μοῦνος / μόνος: The forms in B and V all have ου, with one exception in V (p. 70,8).

νούσημα / νόσημα: This word occurs only once, in the Attic form, as varia lectio for κακόν in B (p. 72,19).

πολύς / πουλύς: Forms of πουλύς occur in V: pp. 84,22; 90,10 πουλῦν; pp. 76,17. 19; 84,25. 26 πουλύ; in B: p. 80,6 πουλυ. These epic forms can be discarded in reconstructing the text.

π- / κ-, ὁπ- / ὁκ-:

In three instances B and V both have π forms: p. 72,6 ὅπῃ; p. 64,17. 20 που. Otherwise B has κ forms, where V uses either short or π forms: p. 78,18 κου; p. 70,24 κως; p. 70,22 ὁκοι; pp. 68,13; 70,11; 78,30; 80,2. 6. 25 ὁκοῖος; pp. 68, 13; 72,17; 74,6. 11; 78,30; 80,17. 21; 84,10 ὁκόσος; p. 70,14 ὁκοσοστισοῦν; pp. 64,18; 70,20; 74,2. 3bis. 4. 16; 76,10 ὁκόταν; p. 74,4 ὁκότερος; pp. 66,8; 70,5 (ὅπη V); 78,27; 80,5 ὅκου; pp. 70,21; 72,18. 20; 78,12 (ὡς V); 84,3 ὅκως; p. 74,18 ὁκωσοῦν.
κ forms are generally considered Ionic; however, we know from Galen that there was variation in this regard in the Hippocratic manuscripts available to him, with Artemidorus Capito using the π forms.[1] Moreover, κ forms are rare in inscriptions, and our earliest manuscripts vary in the usage of κ and π or short forms.[2] Due to the consistent use of π and short forms in V in the text of De capitis vulneribus, three times supported by B, these forms are used throughout in this edition.[3]

σύν / ξύν and συν- / ξυν-:

B and V vary in using σύν (συν-) and ξύν (ξυν-). The preposition occurs in both manuscripts once as σύν (p. 68,18) and once as ξύν (p. 80,20), the prefix as συν- in both manuscripts at pp. 64,24; 76,14, as ξυν- in B and as συν- in V at pp. 64,9; 78,1. It should be noted that in the case of the compounds -φέρειν and -φορή the form ξυμ- occurs with only one exception (p. 90,9) in B and V or in V alone where the text in B is lost. σύν / συν- is used in this edition.

τάμνειν / τέμνειν:

The Ionic α stem is found in both B and V, with one exception in V (p. 80,9 τεμνόμενα).

II. Morphology

1. Nouns

In the o-declension the dat. pl. occurs in the short form only twice in B: p. 72,

[1] See Gal., In Hipp. Epid. VI comm. I 1: CMG V 10,2,2, p. 6,10–14.
[2] Cf. Jouanna, in: CMG I 1,3, pp. 144–145.
[3] Cf. Kühlewein, vol. II, pp. XII–XIII.

14. 28 τοῖς ὀφθαλμοῖς. – The gen. pl. of οὖς is given in both manuscripts as οὐάτων.

ι-stem nouns in B retain the ι in the gen. sing., gen. pl. and acc. pl. with one exception: p. 80,29 ῥηξίων] ριξεων. In V these nouns have in the gen. sing. the ending -ηος with exception of φύσεως at p. 74,1, in the gen. pl. the endings -ηων (pp. 64,31; 78,12) and -εων (p. 80,29, in agreement with B), and in the acc. pl. once the ending -ηας: p. 72,21 φλάσιας] φάσηας. The endings -ηος, -ηων and -ηας in V represent scribal eccentricity rather than transmission of original spellings.[1]

2. Adjectives

In adjectives in -υς the feminine ending -έα (-έη) occurs only in V concerning the word εὐρύς: pp. 68,3; 70,13 εὐρέαι; p. 72,4 εὐρέη (hyperionism; cf. above, pp. 46–47). Since forms in -εῖα prevail in the text of De capitis vulneribus, they are used in this edition.

In V (B deest) the superlative of παχύς occurs once as πάχιστος (p. 90,33), once as παχύτατος (p. 92,5).

πλέος / πλέως:

An example of the ambivalent neuter plural occurs, πλέα (p. 64,7), but also an example of the neuter singular where B has the Ionic πλέον and V has πλέων (p. 84,9).

πολλός / πολύς:

The Ionic form πολλόν occurs unambiguously only in V, once as acc. sing. masc. and once as adverb: p. 84,12–13 ἐπὶ πολλὸν χρόνον V: επι πολλυν χρονον B; p. 78,7 πολλόν τε ἐλασσόνων V: πολλων τε ελασσονων B. In these two cases the Ionic form has been accepted although the form πολύ(ν) is to be found in the text many times.

3. Pronouns and pronominal adjectives with parasitic ε

B and V share three examples of pronouns with hyperionic ε: p. 64,26 αὐτέου; p. 74,18 αὐτέω; p. 84,11 τουτέων. B has, with few exceptions, the artificial forms: p. 62,23 αυτεου; p. 74,18 αυτεω; p. 64,6 αυτεων; p. 82,25 αυτεης; p. 76,14 αὐτεησι; pp. 72,27; 74,2. 9. 24; 76,6 ἑωυτεου; pp. 64,11. 30; 72,25; 80, 26 ἑωυτεω; p. 70,16. 17 ἑωυτεων; p. 84,11 εωυτεηι; p. 62,6 τουτεου; pp. 62, 11. 15; 72,23; 74,8 τουτεω; pp. 64,30; 72,25; 76,7; 78,9; 84,22 τουτεων; p. 70, 11 τοιουτεου; p. 74,27 τοιουτεων.

4. εἶναι

The participle and the subjunctive of εἶναι and ἐνεῖναι have in B and V the forms ἐο-, ἐου-, ἐω- with five exceptions in V (pp. 66,17; 74,25; 82,1 οὖσαι; 88,2. 8). The Ionic forms have been used throughout in this edition.

[1] Cf. Jouanna, in: CMG I 1,3, p. 149.

C. Structure of De capitis vulneribus

The treatise De capitis vulneribus deals exclusively with wounds of the skull. Its material is organized as follows:

Ch. 1: Description of the skull, in particular, the sutures and diploe.

Ch. 2–3: The thickness of the skull and its relation to the degree of injury and the chances of survival after injury.

Ch. 4–8: Types of skull injury: fractures (ch. 4); crush-injury (ch. 5); depressed fracture (ch. 6); hedrē in combination with other injuries and hedrē alone (ch.7); injury elsewhere than the site of trauma (ch. 8).

Ch. 9: Indications for trephination.

Ch. 10–12: Clinical evaluation: examination of wound (ch. 10); relevant history (ch. 11); presence of suture at injury site (ch. 12).

Ch. 13–20: Treatment (use of lint dressings, poultices, bandages; extension of scalp wound by incision; use of blackening agent and rasping; indications for trephination; suppuration and need to keep wound clean and dry; separation of skull fragments; granulation tissue; differences in skulls of children; signs of fatal outcome; significance of facial edema).

Ch. 21: Technique of trephination.

In antiquity the text known to us had already received an extension to its end. The existence of such an addition, only traces of which remain, is attested to by Galen. In his fourth commentary on Regimen in acute diseases he discusses the tendency for material to be added at the end of works and mentions De capitis vulneribus as an example: καὶ μὲν δὴ καὶ ἄλλας ἔστι ῥήσεις εὑρεῖν ἐν τῷ προκειμένῳ βιβλίῳ φανερῶς οὐκ οὔσας ἀξίας Ἱπποκράτους, ὡς ὑπονοῆσαι παρεγγεγράφθαι τοῖς γνησίοις, ὥσπερ γε καὶ κατὰ τοὺς Ἀφορισμοὺς ἐφάνησαν ἔνιοι τοιοῦτοι πρὸς τοῖς τελευταίοις μέρεσι τοῦ βιβλίου. τῷ γὰρ ἐν μνήμῃ πολλοῖς εἶναι τὰ πρῶτα τῶν συγγραμμάτων οἱ παρεγγράφοντες εἰς τὰ τελευταῖα παρεγγράφουσι· τοῦτο γοῦν αὐτὸ καὶ κατὰ τὸ Περὶ τῶν ἐν κεφαλῇ τρωμάτων ἐφάνη γεγονὸς ἔτι τε κατὰ τὸ δεύτερον τῶν Ἐπιδημιῶν. (In Hipp. De victu acut. comm. IV prooem.: CMG V 9,1, p. 271,13–20). The only remnants of this appendix are to be found in Galen's Hippocratic Lexicon: ἐκλουέσθω· σημαίνει ποτὲ καὶ τὸ προσκλυζέσθω, ὡς ἐν τῷ Περὶ ἀφόρων καὶ τοῖς προσκειμένοις τοῖς Περὶ τῶν ἐν κεφαλῇ τρωμάτων (Ling. s. dict. exolet. Hipp. explic.: XIX 95,9–11 K.), and: σφάκερος· ἐν τοῖς προσκειμένοις τοῖς Περὶ τῶν ἐν τῇ κεφαλῇ τρωμάτων· «κεφαλαλγία δὲ καὶ σφάκερος ἦν ᾖ, κρόμμυα πολέμιον.» ἔν τε τοῖς πλείστοις ἄντικρυς σφαλερὸς γράφεται (ibid.: XIX 144,4–7 K.).

D. De capitis vulneribus and its place in medical literature

I. Vestige of an ancient tradition

De capitis vulneribus, as seen from the nature of its advice, must represent the distillation of generations of surgical experience. It certainly represents one small fragment that has survived from an even more ancient tradition. Another fragment of that tradition is the Edwin Smith papyrus[1], from the 17th c. B.C. and containing material dated, on the basis of its vocabulary, to the early part of the Old Kingdom, 3000–2800 B.C. The Egyptian document displays a number of characteristics seen also in De capitis vulneribus: 1. rational organization of material, 2. accurate clinical observations, 3. association of neurological dysfunction with head injury, 4. development and use of medical terms, and 5. reliance on long-established empirical traditions.

Greek admiration of Egyptian medical practice is expressed by Homer (Od. IV 227–232) and attested by Herodotus (II 84; III 129,2). And the Greek medical centers, which seem to have developed first at the periphery of the Greek world (South Italy, Cyrene, Cos, Cnidus), could scarcely have escaped Egyptian influence. It seems likely that a long-standing exchange of medical ideas, practices, herbs and physicians existed along the Aegean-Mediterranean trade routes. As testimony to what must have been a rich surgical tradition we possess only the Edwin Smith papyrus and, over two millennia later, a few treatises, preserved as part of the Hippocratic Corpus.

II. Date of composition

The treatise De capitis vulneribus belongs thematically to the group of surgical writings handed down in the Hippocratic Corpus and assumed to have originated in the time of Hippocrates. Its subject is skull injuries and, like the other treatises dealing with injuries to bone, it contains practical surgical advice, based on experience and delivered with a strongly empirical tone. The language of the treatise is clear expository prose. As in other early texts of the Corpus Hippocraticum, there is considerable repetition, of words, phrases, and sentences, almost as though the author were intent on emphasizing his points by repetition, but otherwise he is not verbose.[2] There is no use of rhetorical devices. The vocabulary is basic and simple. Grammar and syntax are standard. The infinitive is used commonly for the imperative, as in many Hippocratic writings. The language, therefore, and the content of De capitis vulneribus are compatible with a date of composition around 400 B.C.

External evidence for the date of composition comes from two sources. Erotian (Voc. Hipp. collect. B 8: p. 28,10–14 Nachmanson), in his discussion of βλιχῶδες, claimed to be the original reading for γλισχρῶδες, the form transmitted in De capitis vulneribus (p. 88,6), refers to the early third c. Hippocratic Glossary of Bacchius, who considered the word to be πλιχῶδες and gave it a definition that does not accord well with its context in De capitis vulneribus. But if the word discussed was in fact taken from De capitis vulneribus then it must be assumed that enough time had elapsed between the composition of this treatise and Bacchius' Glossary for the term to have become generally unintelligible and possibly also for a generation or two of scribal errors.

1 J. H. Breasted, The Edwin Smith surgical papyrus, 2 vols., Chicago, 1930.

2 Cf. Withington, in: Hippocrates, p. 5 and p. 91, with reference to De fracturis and De articulis.

Another indicator for dating is found in similarities of wording between our text and the fifth book of Epidemics:

p. 78,1–2 συγκλέπτουσι γὰρ τὴν γνώμην καὶ τὴν ὄψιν τοῦ ἰητροῦ αὗται αἱ ῥαφαὶ ...; cf. Epid. V 27: V 226,11 L.: ἔκλεψαν δέ μου τὴν γνώμην αἱ ῥαφαὶ ...

pp. 86,35–88,2 ὁπόταν τις ... ἁμάρτῃ καὶ μήτε ξύσῃ μήτε πρίσῃ †μήτε δεόμενον ...; cf. Epid. V 27: V 226,10 L.: Τοῦτο παρέλαθέ με δεόμενον πρισθῆναι· ...; 28: 226,20 L.: Τοῦτο ἐγνώσθη ὀρθῶς πρίσεως δεόμενον· ...

p. 88,13–14 ἢν δ' ἐν τῷ ἐπὶ δεξιὰ τῆς κεφαλῆς ἔχῃ τὸ ἕλκος, τὰ ἐπ' ἀριστερὰ τοῦ σώματος ὁ σπασμὸς ἐπιλαμβάνει.; cf. Epid. V 28: V 228,2–4 L.: σπασμὸς δὲ χεῖρα τὴν ἀριστερὴν ἐπελάμβανεν· ἐν γὰρ τοῖσι δεξιοῖσι μᾶλλον εἶχε τὸ ἕλκος.

p. 88,25 καὶ εἴ τις ἅπτοιτο τοῦ οἰδήματος, ὀδυνῷτο ⟨ἄν⟩ ...; cf. Epid. V 16: V 216,3 L.: καὶ ὠδυνᾶτο τὸ οἴδημα· ...

These statements in Epidemics V, which occur in the context of case histories, certainly bring to mind the pronouncements of De capitis vulneribus. There knowledge gained in practice is distilled into generalized advice for the treatment of various types of head injury; in Epidemics V this general advice is applied to individual cases. Accordingly, it is reasonable to assume that the author of Epidemics V knew the text of De capitis vulneribus, and this relationship should provide a further terminus ante quem for its composition. One difficulty, however, for precise dating is that views concerning the time of composition of Epidemics V differ. The latest estimate, advocated by V. Langholf, places its date of composition no earlier than 336 B.C.[1] It is plausible then to conclude from this external evidence that De capitis vulneribus existed and was well known by the mid-fourth century.

III. Relationship to other works of the Corpus Hippocraticum and to later medical authors

De capitis vulneribus is not named in any Hippocratic treatise; however, there are similarities in content and expression, which show that there exists a more or less tight web of relationships between this text and others in the Hippocratic Corpus.

Of all the Hippocratic treatises De ulceribus resembles De capitis vulneribus the most, both in substance (a shared concern for the dryness of wounds) and language. The most marked resemblances are the following:

p. 66,6–7 ἐν χειμῶνι πλείονα χρόνον ζῇ ὤνθρωπος ἢ ἐν θέρει, ...; cf. De ulc.

1 See V. Langholf, Syntaktische Untersuchungen zu Hippokrates-Texten. Brachylogische Syntagmen in den individuellen Krankheits-Fallbeschreibungen der hippokratischen Schriftensammlung, Wiesbaden, 1977, S. 15–17, with discussion of other datings (375–350 or 360–350 B.C.).

5: VI 404,21–22 L.: Ἕλκεσι τοῖσι πλείστοισιν ὥρη ἡ θερμοτέρη ξυμφορωτέρη τοῦ χειμῶνος, πλὴν τοῖσιν ἐν κεφαλῇ καὶ κοιλίῃ, ...

p. 78,13–15 ἕλκος ἐν κεφαλῇ οὐ χρὴ τέγγειν οὐδενί, οὐδὲ οἴνῳ, ἄλλως ἥκιστα· οὐδὲ καταπλάσσειν ..., οὐδ' ἐπιδεῖν χρὴ ἕλκος ἐν κεφαλῇ, ...; cf. De ulc. 1: VI 400,2–6 L.: Ἕλκεα ξύμπαντα οὐ χρὴ τέγγειν, πλὴν οἴνῳ ... Ἀνεπίδετον δὲ ἐᾶν ἄμεινόν ἐστιν, ὅ τι γε μὴ καταπλάσσεται· οὐδὲ καταπλάσσειν ἐνδεχόμενόν ἐστιν ἔνια τῶν ἑλκέων, ...

p. 80,6–8 τὰ κυκλοτερέα τῶν ἑλκέων καὶ ὑπόκοιλα ... ἐπανατάμνων τὸν κύκλον διχῇ κατὰ μῆκος, ὥσπερ πέφυκεν ὥνθρωπος, μακρὸν ποιεῖν τὸ ἕλκος; cf. De ulc. 8: VI 406,10–13 L.: Τῶν ἑλκέων τὰ κυκλοτερέα ἢν ὑπόκοιλα ᾖ, ἐν κύκλῳ πάντη ἐπιτάμνειν χρὴ ... κατὰ μῆκος τῆς φύσιος τοῦ ἀνθρώπου.

p. 82,16 ὑποτείνας ὀθόνιον ἐλαίῳ τέγξας, εἶτα καταπλάσας ...; cf. De ulc. 11: VI 410,20–21 L.: καταπλάσσειν, ὀθόνιον ὑποτείνας λεπτὸν καθαρόν, οἴνῳ καὶ ἐλαίῳ τέγξας ...

p. 84,13–16 ἀλλὰ χρὴ διάπυον μὲν ποιῆσαι τὸ ἕλκος ὡς τάχιστα. οὕτως γὰρ ἂν ἥκιστα φλεγμαίνοι τὰ περιέχοντα τὸ ἕλκος ... ἀνάγκη γὰρ ἔχει τὰς σάρκας τὰς κοπείσας καὶ φλασθείσας ὑπὸ τοῦ βέλεος ὑποπύους γενομένας ἐκτακῆναι (pp. 74,29–76,1 ἀνάγκη γὰρ τὰς σάρκας τὰς φλασθείσας καὶ κοπείσας πύος γενομένας ἐκτακῆναι); cf. De ulc. 1: VI 400,16–17; 402, 7–11 L.: Τὰ δὲ νεότρωτα ἕλκεα πάντα ἥκιστα ἂν φλεγμήναιεν αὐτά τε καὶ τὰ περιέχοντα, εἴ τις διαπυΐσκοι ὡς τάχιστα ... Ἤ τις δ' ὑπὸ τοῦ βέλεος ἐφλάσθη καὶ ἐκόπη σάρξ, ταύτην δὲ ἰητρεύειν, ὅκως διάπυος ὡς τάχιστα γένηται· ἧσσόν τε γὰρ φλεγμαίνει· καὶ ἀνάγκη τὰς σάρκας τὰς φλασθείσας καὶ κοπείσας σαπείσας καὶ πῦον γενομένας ἐκτακῆναι ...

p. 84,16–19 ἐπειδὰν δὲ καθαρθῇ ... καὶ οὕτως οὐκ ἂν ὑπερσαρκήσειε τὸ ἕλκος; cf. De ulc. 6: VI 404,24–25 L.: Τὰ ἕλκεα ὁκόσα μὴ καλῶς καθαρθέντα ... ταῦτα ὑπερσαρκέει μάλιστα ...

p. 90,3–4 τούτου χρὴ τὴν κάτω κοιλίην ὑποκαθῆραι φαρμάκῳ ...; cf. De ulc. 3: VI 404,11–12 L.: Ὑποκάθαρσις τῆς κάτω κοιλίης ξυμφέρει τοῖσι πλείστοισι τῶν ἑλκέων καὶ ἐν τρώμασιν ἐν κεφαλῇ ἐοῦσι ...

These similarities are marked enough to suggest either a common author or direct use of one treatise in the composition of the other.

Analogies to facts described in De capitis vulneribus are also found in the treatises Coan Prenotions, Places in Man, Prorrhetic II, Aphorisms and Fractures;[1] however, no definite conclusions can be drawn concerning the nature of the dependence.

p. 80,10–14 ὁ δὲ κρόταφος ... τοῦτο δὲ τὸ χωρίον μὴ τάμνειν. σπασμὸς γὰρ ἐπιλαμβάνει τὸν τμηθέντα. καὶ ἢν μὲν ἐν τῷ ἐπ' ἀριστερὰ τμηθῇ κροτάφῳ, τὰ ἐπὶ δεξιὰ ὁ σπασμὸς ἐπιλαμβάνει, ἢν δ' ⟨ἐν τῷ⟩ ἐπὶ δεξιὰ τμηθῇ κροτάφῳ, τὰ ἐπ' ἀριστερὰ ὁ σπασμὸς ἐπιλαμβάνει; cf. Coac. praenot. 488:

[1] Epidemics V also belongs to this group of treatises; see above, p. 53.

V 696,1–2 L.: Ὁκόσοισι κρόταφος τάμνεται, σπασμὸς ἐκ τῶν ἐναντίων τῆς τομῆς ἐπιγίνεται.

p. 74,3–4. 16–17. 23–26 ὅταν ἐξ ὑψηλοτέρου ... μᾶλλον ἢ ὅταν ἐξ ἰσοπέδου τοῦ χωρίου ... καὶ κατ' ἀντίον γένηται τὸ ὀστέον τοῦ βέλεος ... Τῶν δὲ βελέων ῥήγνυσι μάλιστα τὸ ὀστέον ... τὰ στρογγύλα ... ἐόντα ... βαρέα ...; cf. Coac. praenot. 491: V 696,8–10 L.: ῥήγνυται (sc. τὰ ἐν κεφαλῇ ὀστέα) δὲ ὑπὸ τῶν βαρέων καὶ στρογγύλων βελέων μάλιστα, καὶ ἐκ τῶν ἐξ ὑπεναντίου φερομένων, καὶ μὴ ἐξ ἰσοπέδου.

p. 76,17–19 καὶ γίνεται καὶ αὐτὴ ἡ ῥῆξις χαλεπωτέρη φράσασθαι ἐρρωγότος τοῦ ὀστέου, διὰ τοῦτο, ὅτι κατ' αὐτὴν τὴν ῥαφὴν ἡ ῥῆξις γίνεται ...; cf. Coac. praenot. 491: V 696,7–8 L.: Τῶν ῥηγνυμένων ἐν κεφαλῇ ὀστέων, χαλεπώτατον γνῶναι τὰ κατὰ τὰς ῥαφὰς ῥηγνύμενα ...

p. 84,20–23 ἢν γὰρ αὐτίκα ἐκπρίσας τὸ ὀστέον καὶ ἀφελὼν ἀπὸ τῆς μήνιγγος ψιλώσῃς, αὐτὴν καθαρὴν χρὴ ποιῆσαι ὡς τάχιστα καὶ ξηρήν, ὡς μὴ ἐπὶ πολὺν χρόνον ὑγρὴ ἐοῦσα μυδᾷ τε καὶ ξαίνηται· τούτων γὰρ οὕτως γινομένων σαπῆναι αὐτὴν κίνδυνος; cf. De locis in hom. 32: VI 324,7–9 L.: ἢν δὲ ῥαγῇ (sc. τὸ ὀστέον) καὶ ῥωγμὴ ἐγγένηται, ἐπικίνδυνον· τοῦτον πρίειν, ὡς μὴ κατὰ τὴν ῥωγμὴν τοῦ ὀστέου ἰχὼρ ῥέων τὴν μήνιγγα σήπῃ ...

p. 76,6–9 Ἀλλὰ χρὴ ... ἐρώτησιν ποιεῖσθαι ... ἢν ὁ τρωθεὶς καρωθῇ ... καὶ πέσῃ. (p. 82,12–13 ἐκαρώθη καὶ κατέπεσεν); cf. Prorrh. II 14: IX 38,4–6 L.: Πυνθάνεσθαι δὲ χρὴ ἐπὶ πᾶσι τοῖσιν ἀξίοις λόγου τρώμασιν ... εἰ ... κατέπεσεν ὥνθρωπος, ἢ εἰ ἐκαρώθη ...

p. 88,23 ἐψιλωμένου δὲ τοῦ ὀστέου οἴδημα ἐπιγένηται ἐρυθρὸν καὶ ἐρυσιπελατῶδες ...; cf. Aphor. VII 19: IV 582,4 L.: Ἐπὶ ὀστέου ψιλώσει, ἐρυσίπελας.

p. 84,13–15. 17–18 ἀλλὰ χρὴ διάπυον μὲν ποιῆσαι τὸ ἕλκος ὡς τάχιστα. οὕτως γὰρ ... τάχιστ' ἂν καθαρὸν εἴη ... οὕτως γὰρ ἂν τάχιστα ὑγιὲς γένοιτο ξηρῆς σαρκὸς βλαστούσης ... (p. 86,10 ἐπανέρχεται [sc. τὰ ὀστέα] δὲ τῆς σαρκὸς ὑποφυομένης); cf. De fract. 33: II 98,1–6 Kw. = III 534,1–4 L.: ὡς μὲν οὖν τὸ ἐπίπαν τάχιστα τούτων ὀστέα ἀφίσταται, ὧν τάχισται μὲν αἱ ἐκπυήσιες, τάχισται δὲ καὶ κάλλισται αἱ σαρκοφυίαι· καὶ γὰρ αἱ ὑποφυόμεναι σάρκες κατὰ τὸ σιναρὸν αὗται μετεωρίζουσιν τὰ ὀστέα ὡς ἐπὶ τὸ πολύ.

As part of the Hippocratic Corpus De capitis vulneribus undoubtedly constituted a primary reference work and a basis for development in the management of head injuries. Unfortunately Hellenistic literature on the subject has not survived, preventing an assessment of the extent and degree of its influence in Greek antiquity. But Galen's statements about De capitis vulneribus and his attention to it confirm its importance as late as the 2nd c. A.D. (see above, pp. 36–39; 51).

Other late authors, however, show little evidence of its influence. Celsus (1st c. A.D.), Heliodorus (1st/2nd c. A.D.) and Paul of Aegina (7th c. A.D.) never mention it by name. Celsus devotes the first sections of Book VIII of his Medicina (Med. VIII 1,1–4; 3–4: CML I, pp. 363,3–364,6; 374,23–382,16) to a discussion of the skull and its pathology. Some of the points made correspond to those of De capitis vulneribus: attention to symptoms, the type of weapon, the use of a probe, the difficulty distinguishing skull sutures from fractures, the need to open the wound if it does not allow proper inspection of the bone, the use of a black solution to identify fractures, fractures occurring elsewhere than the site of impact, and the growth of "new tissue". But all of these points could have been part of standard management and not specifically derived from De capitis vulneribus. And the differences in anatomical description, diagnosis and treatment in the two works are substantial: cranial sutures are described differently; classification of the types of head injury is minimal in Celsus' Medicina and largely ignores two of the major categories of De capitis vulneribus; the author of De capitis vulneribus recommends surgery for linear fractures but not for depressed fractures while Celsus advises just the opposite; and details of surgical technique differ considerably. In this part of his work Celsus mentions Hippocrates only once by name, recounting that Hippocrates described how he had failed to recognize a fracture because it occurred at the site of a cranial suture (Med. VIII 4,3–4: CML I, p. 378,3–11). There is a general discussion of this problem in De capitis vulneribus (12,3: p. 78,1–3) but Celsus is undoubtedly referring here to the clinical case reported in Epidemics V 27 (V 226,10–12 L.). And the fact that Celsus concedes that he introduced the account primarily to recall "the great teacher" suggests that De capitis vulneribus did not serve as a basis for this section of his work.

Heliodorus, like Celsus, presents some advice similar to that in De capitis vulneribus, but nothing, in wording or content, to suggest direct use of the treatise (see Orib., Coll. med. rel. XLVI 7–19: CMG VI 2,1, pp. 216,27–226, 28).

The advice on the treatment of head injuries given by Paul of Aegina differs considerably from that of De capitis vulneribus and in his discussions of head injury he does not refer to De capitis vulneribus by title. However, in these discussions he twice refers to Hippocrates. The first reference occurs in a section on removal of weapons, εἰ δὲ κεκρυμμένον (sc. τὸ βέλος), δεῖ, φησὶν Ἱπποκράτης, εἰ μὲν δύναιτο ὁ τρωθείς, ἐπ' ἐκείνου τοῦ σχήματος αὐτὸν ποιήσαντα σημειώσασθαι, ἐφ' οὗ καὶ τιτρωσκόμενος ἐτύγχανεν, εἰ δὲ μὴ δύναιτο, κείμενον γοῦν ὡς οἷόν τε κατ' ἐκεῖνο σχηματίσαντες τῇ μηλώσει χρησόμεθα (VI 88,3: CMG IX 2, p. 131,6–10). If Paul had De capitis vulneribus in mind here, the reference would be to the short passage, ἀλλ' ἕδρην τε τοῦ βέλεος ἐλέγχει μήλωσις (10,4: p. 72,26).

The other reference is clearly to a statement in ch. 20 of De capitis vulneribus. In discussing a febrile complication of head wounds, the author of De capitis vulneribus says, τούτου χρὴ τὴν κάτω κοιλίην ὑποκαθῆραι φαρμάκῳ, ὅ τι χολὴν ἄγει ... (20,1: p. 90,3–4). Paul, in a similar context, says, ἐπιμενούσης δὲ τῆς φλεγμονῆς (sc. τῆς μήνιγγος) καὶ μηδενὸς ἑτέρου κωλύοντος καὶ χολαγωγῷ φαρμάκῳ καθαίρειν αὐτοὺς Ἱπποκράτης παρακελεύεται (VI 90,9: CMG IX 2, p. 142,20–22).

The advice regarding management of the various types of head injury differs from one to another of these four late writers, and each of them, including Galen, differs from the advice in De capitis vulneribus. It would have been surprising indeed if physicians in antiquity, with no diagnostic aids, and therefore no secure basis for treatment, had agreed on treatment guidelines for head injury cases. That a few procedures remained the same from the time of De capitis vulneribus through that of Celsus and even of Paul of Aegina may reflect general acceptance of some of the less invasive procedures (questioning the patient, enlarging the wound, applying a black solution, giving a purgative) rather than use of the Hippocratic treatise. Still, in a field where no physician could possibly earn a reputation as a great healer, the need to be associated with established surgical tradition would have been strong. Surely Galen and Paul of Aegina, while presenting the surgical advice that seemed best to them, still claimed the security of a long-established surgical tradition, Galen by "defining" the advice of the Hippocratic author (ὅσα τε ἀδιορίστως εἶπε διοριζόμεθα, Meth. med. VI 6: X 444,18 K.), Paul by quoting the master.

IV. Longevity of De capitis vulneribus as a medical text

Following the Latin translations of Calvus in 1525 and Vidius in 1544 De capitis vulneribus became widely available to the Western medical world. Aside from the numerous translations and commentaries (see above, pp. 44–46), references to it occurred in the writings of leading surgeons, e.g. J. Daleschamps (Chirurgie françoise, Lyon, 1573, pp. 635; 668–701), Sir Percival Pott (Observations on the nature and consequences of those injuries to which the head is liable from external violence, London, 1768) and Littré, in the preface to his edition of Hippocrates, states, "Mon but a été de mettre les œuvres hippocratiques complètement à la portée des médecins de notre temps, . . ." (vol. I, p. IX). That any work could remain useful to practising physicians over a period of two and a half millennia is difficult to comprehend for modern physicians, struggling to made adequate use of rapidly improving technologies. But, in the context of pre-twentieth century medicine and given the knowledge available to its author, De capitis vulneribus is a fine example of a practical surgical handbook.

ΙΠΠΟΚΡΑΤΟΥΣ

ΠΕΡΙ ΤΩΝ ΕΝ ΚΕΦΑΛΗΙ ΤΡΩΜΑΤΩΝ

HIPPOCRATES

ON HEAD WOUNDS

CONSPECTVS SIGLORVM ET COMPENDIORVM

B	= Laurentianus Gr. 74,7; s. X
B^2, B^3	= eiusdem codicis correctores
V	= Vaticanus Gr. 276; s. XII

Raro citantur:

N	= Parisinus Gr. 2248; s. XVI
P	= Palatinus Gr. 192; s. XV
C	= Parisinus Gr. 2146; s. XVI
Ho	= Holkhamensis Gr. 92; s. XVI
Ho^2	= eiusdem codicis corrector
E	= Parisinus Gr. 2255; s. XVI
recc.	= codices recentiores

Ald.	= editio Aldina, Venetiis, a. 1526
Frob.	= editio Frobeniana, Basileae, a. 1538
Foes.	= A. Foesius, Magni Hippocratis . . . Opera omnia, Francofurti, a. 1595
Maniaud	= E. Maniaud, Hippocratis Coi Chirurgia, Lutetiae Parisiorum, a. 1619
Lind.	= J. A. van der Linden, Hippocratis Coi . . . Opera omnia, Lugduni Batavorum, a. 1665
Littré	= E. Littré, Œuvres complètes d'Hippocrate, Lutetiae Parisiorum, a. 1841
Erm.	= F. Z. Ermerins, Hippocratis . . . reliquiae, Traiecti ad Rhenum, a. 1859
Reinh.	= K. H. Th. Reinhold, Ἱπποκράτης κομιδῇ, Athenis, a. 1865
Petrequin	= J. E. Petrequin, Chirurgie d'Hippocrate, Lutetiae Parisiorum, a. 1877
Kühlewein	= H. Kühlewein, Hippocratis Opera, Lipsiae, a. 1902
Withington	= E. T. Withington, Hippocrates with an English translation, Londinii et Cantabrigiae, Mass., a. 1928

Corn.	= Cornarius in editionis Aldinae exemplari suo nunc bibliothecae universitatis Goettingensis proprio

Scal.	= emendationes J. J. Scaligeri in editione Hippocratis . . . De capitis vulneribus libri a F. Vertuniano curata, Lutetiae Parisiorum, a. 1578, typis expressae
Portus	= emendationes Ae. Porti in editione Foesii typis expressae
Mart.	= emendationes J. Martini in editione Foesii, col. 252sq., typis expressae

ΙΠΠΟΚΡΑΤΟΥΣ

ΠΕΡΙ ΤΩΝ ΕΝ ΚΕΦΑΛΗΙ ΤΡΩΜΑΤΩΝ

III 182 L. 1. Τῶν ἀνθρώπων αἱ κεφαλαὶ οὐδὲν ὁμοίως σφίσιν αὐταῖς οὐδὲ αἱ
II 1 Kw. ῥαφαὶ τῆς κεφαλῆς πάντων κατὰ ταὐτὰ πεφύκασιν. ἀλλ' ὅστις μὲν ἔχει ἐκ
τοῦ ἔμπροσθεν τῆς κεφαλῆς προβολήν – ἡ δὲ προβολή ἐστι τὸ τοῦ ὀστέου
ἐξέχον στρογγύλον παρὰ τὸ ἄλλο –, τούτου εἰσὶν αἱ ῥαφαὶ πεφυκυῖαι ἐν
τῇ κεφαλῇ, ὥσπερ γράμμα τὸ ταῦ γράφεται. τὴν μὲν γὰρ βραχυτέρην
γραμμὴν ἔχει πρὸ τῆς προβολῆς ἐπικαρσίην πεφυκυῖαν, τὴν δ' ἑτέρην, μα-
κροτέρην γραμμὴν ἔχει διὰ μέσης τῆς κεφαλῆς κατὰ μῆκος πεφυκυῖαν πρὸς
2 τὸν τράχηλον αἰεί. ὅστις δ' ὄπισθεν τῆς κεφαλῆς τὴν προβολὴν ἔχει, αἱ ῥα-
φαὶ τούτῳ πεφύκασι τὰ ἐναντία ἢ τῷ προτέρῳ. ἡ μὲν γὰρ βραχυτέρη
γραμμὴ πρὸ τῆς προβολῆς πέφυκεν ἐπικαρσίη, ἡ δὲ μακροτέρη γραμμὴ διὰ
3 μέσης τῆς κεφαλῆς πέφυκε κατὰ μῆκος ἐς τὸ μέτωπον αἰεί. ὅστις δὲ ἀμφοτέ-
184 ρωθεν τῆς κεφαλῆς προβολὴν ἔχει, ἔκ τε τοῦ ἔμπροσθεν καὶ | ἐκ τοῦ ὄπι-
2 σθεν, τούτῳ αἱ ῥαφαί εἰσιν / ὁμοίως πεφυκυῖαι, ὡς γράμμα τὸ ἦτα γράφε-
ται. πεφύκασι δὲ τῶν γραμμέων αἱ μὲν μακραὶ πρὸ τῆς προβολῆς ἑκατέρης
ἐπικάρσιαι πεφυκυῖαι, ἡ δὲ βραχεῖα διὰ μέσης τῆς κεφαλῆς κατὰ μῆκος
4 πρὸς ἑκατέρην τελευτῶσα τῇσι μακρῇσι γραμμῇσιν. ὅστις δὲ μηδετέρωθι
μηδεμίαν προβολὴν ἔχει, οὗτος ἔχει τὰς ῥαφὰς τῆς κεφαλῆς, ὡς γράμμα τὸ
χεῖ γράφεται. πεφύκασι δὲ αἱ γραμμαὶ ἡ μὲν ἑτέρη ἐπικαρσίη πρὸς τὸν
κρόταφον ἀφήκουσα, ἡ δ' ἑτέρη κατὰ μῆκος διὰ μέσης τῆς κεφαλῆς.
5 Διπλόον δέ ἐστι τὸ ὀστέον κατὰ μέσην τὴν κεφαλήν. σκληρότατον δὲ
καὶ πυκνότατον αὐτοῦ πέφυκε τό τε ἀνώτατον, ἡ ὁμόχροια τοῦ ὀστέου ἡ
186 ὑπὸ τῇ σαρκί, | καὶ τὸ κατώτατον τὸ πρὸς τῇ μήνιγγι, ἡ ὁμόχροια τοῦ
ὀστέου ἡ κάτω· ἀποχωρέον δὲ ἀπὸ τοῦ ἀνωτάτου ὀστέου καὶ τοῦ κατω-
τάτου, ἀπὸ τῶν σκληροτάτων καὶ πυκνοτάτων, ἐπὶ τὸ μαλθακώτερον καὶ

3sq. οὐδὲ – πεφύκασιν] *cf.* Cels. Med. VIII 1,2: CML I, p. 363,12sq. Plat. Tim. 76 a Arist. Hist. anim. I 7; III 7: 491 b 2–5; 516 a 15–20 8 ἐπικαρσίην] *cf.* Erot. Voc. Hipp. collect. E 64: p. 40,13 Nachmanson 23 ὁμόχροια] *cf.* Hipp. De fract. 2: II 47,12 Kw. = III 418,5 L. De carn. 17,4: p. 18,10 Deichgräber = VIII 606,16 L.

1 Ἱπποκράτους *om.* V 3 φησὶν B 5 τὸ] αὐτέου B 6 *post* τούτου *add.* τέ B, δ' V: *corr. Ald.* 7 ὡς V 8 μακροτέρην *om.* V 9 πεφυκυῖαν *om.* V πρὸς] ἐς V 11 τουτέων B²: τούτων V: τούτου Ho τἀναντία V ἢ *om.* B 12 πρὸ *om.* B γραμμὴ^{II} *om.* V 13 *post* δὲ *add.* καὶ V 14 ἐκ *om.* V 16 γραμμάτων V ἑκατεραι B: ἑκατέρη V: *corr. Ald.* 17 ἐπικάρσιοι V 18 τὴν μακρὴν γραμμήν *Ald.* δὲ *om.* V 21 ἀφηκουσαν B: *corr.* N: ἀφίκουσαι V 23 τε *om.* V ἡ^{I}] ἦν B: ἣ ἡ N ἡ^{II} *om.* V 24 μήνιγγι] μηνιγγιηι B, *in* μήνιγγι, ἧι *mut.* B²: μήνιγγι, ᾗ N 26 μαλθακότατον B

HIPPOCRATES

ON HEAD WOUNDS

1. The heads of men are not all alike, nor are the cranial sutures arranged the same in all. He who has a prominence at the front of his head – a prominence is a rounded projection of the bone beyond the other (bone) – has his cranial sutures arranged as the letter *tau* (T) is written. For he has the shorter line situated transversely above the prominence, and the other, longer line situated longitudinally through the middle of the skull, extending invaria-
bly to the neck. But he who has the prominence at the back of his head has 2
his sutures arranged the reverse of the former. For the shorter line is situated
transversely above the prominence, and the longer line is situated longitudi-
nally through the middle of the skull extending invariably to the forehead.
And he who has a prominence at both ends of his head, both front and back, 3
in the same manner has his sutures arranged as the letter *eta* (H) is written.
The long lines are situated transversely above each prominence, and the short
line longitudinally through the middle of the skull (extending) in the direc-
tion of each (prominence and) terminating in the long lines. But he who has 4
no prominence at either end has his cranial sutures as the letter *chi* (X) is
written. The lines are situated, one transversely extending to the temple (on
either side), the other longitudinally through the middle of the skull.

The bone of the midpart of the skull is double. The hardest and densest 5
part of it is both the outermost, the even surface of the bone just under the scalp, and the innermost, the even undersurface of the bone, next to the membrane (dura mater); passing from the outermost and innermost layers the bone always goes from the hardest and densest parts to the softer, less dense and

ἧσσον πυκνὸν καὶ ἐπικοιλότερον ἐς τὴν διπλόην αἰεί. ἡ δὲ διπλόη κοιλότα-
188 6 τον καὶ μαλθακώτατον καὶ | μάλιστα σηραγγῶδές ἐστιν. ἔστι δὲ καὶ πᾶν
3 τὸ ὀστέον τῆς κεφαλῆς πλὴν / κάρτα ὀλίγου, τοῦ τε ἀνωτάτου καὶ τοῦ
κατωτάτου, σπόγγῳ ὅμοιον, καὶ ἔχει τὸ ὀστέον ἐν ἑωυτῷ ὅμοια σαρκία
πολλὰ καὶ ὑγρά, καὶ εἴ τις αὐτὰ διατρίβοι τοῖσι δακτύλοισιν, αἷμα ἂν
διαγίνοιτο ἐξ αὐτῶν. ἔνεστι δ' ἐν τῷ ὀστέῳ καὶ φλέβια λεπτότερα καὶ κοι-
λότερα αἵματος πλέα. σκληρότητος μέν νυν καὶ μαλθακότητος καὶ κοιλό-
τητος ὧδε ἔχει.

2. Παχύτητι δὲ καὶ λεπτότητι συμπάσης τῆς κεφαλῆς τὸ ὀστέον λε-
πτότατόν ἐστι καὶ ἀσθενέστατον τὸ κατὰ βρέγμα, καὶ σάρκα ὀλιγίστην
καὶ λεπτοτάτην ἔχει ἐπὶ ἑωυτῷ ταύτῃ τῆς κεφαλῆς τὸ ὀστέον, καὶ ὁ ἐγκέ-
2 φαλος κατὰ τοῦτο τῆς κεφαλῆς πλεῖστος ὕπεστιν. καὶ δὴ ὅτι οὕτως ταῦτα
190 ἔχει, τῶν τε τρω|σίων καὶ τῶν βελέων ἴσων τε ἐόντων κατὰ μέγεθος καὶ
ἐλασσόνων καὶ ὁμοίως τε τρωθεὶς καὶ ἧσσον, τὸ ὀστέον ταύτῃ τῆς κεφαλῆς
φλᾶταί τε μᾶλλον καὶ ῥήγνυται καὶ ἔσω ἐσφλᾶται, καὶ θανασιμώτερά
ἐστι καὶ χαλεπώτερα ἰητρεύεσθαί τε καὶ ἐκφυγγάνειν τὸν θάνατον ταύτῃ
ἤ που ἄλλοθι τῆς κεφαλῆς. ἐξίσων τε ἐόντων τῶν τρωμάτων ⟨. . .⟩ καὶ ὁμοί-
ως τε τρωθεὶς καὶ ἧσσον, ἀποθνήσκει ὁ ἄνθρωπος, ὅταν καὶ ἄλλως μέλλῃ
4 ἀποθανεῖσθαι ἐκ τοῦ τρώματος, ἐν ἐλάσσονι χρόνῳ ὁ / ταύτῃ ἔχων τὸ
3 τρῶμα τῆς κεφαλῆς ἤ που ἄλλοθι. ὁ γὰρ ἐγκέφαλος τάχιστά τε καὶ μάλι-
στα κατὰ τὸ βρέγμα αἰσθάνεται τῶν κακῶν τῶν γινομένων ἔν τε τῇ σαρκὶ
καὶ τῷ ὀστέῳ· ὑπὸ λεπτοτάτῳ γὰρ ὀστέῳ ἐστὶ ταύτῃ ὁ ἐγκέφαλος καὶ
4 ὀλιγίστῃ σαρκί, καὶ ὁ πλεῖστος ἐγκέφαλος ὑπὸ τῷ βρέγματι κεῖται. τῶν
δὲ ἄλλων τὸ κατὰ τοὺς κροτάφους ἀσθενέστατόν ἐστι. συμβολή τε γὰρ
τῆς κάτω γνάθου πρὸς τὸ κρανίον καὶ κίνησις ἔνεστιν ἐν τῷ κροτάφῳ ἄνω
καὶ κάτω ὥσπερ ἄρθρου. καὶ ἡ ἀκοὴ πλησίον γίνεται αὐτοῦ· καὶ φλὲψ διὰ
τοῦ κροτάφου τέταται κοίλη τε καὶ ἰσχυρή.
5 Ἰσχυρότερον δ' ἐστὶ τῆς κεφαλῆς τὸ ὀστέον ἅπαν τὸ ὄπισθεν τῆς κο-
192 ρυφῆς καὶ τῶν | οὐάτων ἢ ἅπαν τὸ πρόσθεν· καὶ σάρκα πλείονα καὶ βαθυ-
6 τέρην ἐπὶ ἑωυτῷ ἔχει τοῦτο τὸ ὀστέον. καὶ δὴ τούτων οὕτως ἐχόντων ὑπό
τε τῶν τρωσίων καὶ τῶν βελέων ἴσων ἐόντων καὶ ὁμοίων καὶ μεζόνων καὶ
[μειόνων] ὁμοίως τιτρωσκόμενος καὶ μᾶλλον, ταύτῃ τῆς κεφαλῆς τὸ ὀστέον
ἧσσον ῥήγνυται καὶ φλᾶται ἔσω. κἢν μέλλῃ ὥνθρωπος ἀποθνήσκειν καὶ

1 διπλόην] *cf.* Ruf. De corp. hum. part. appellat. 135: p. 151,6sq. D.-R. 28–29 οὐάτων] *cf.* Cels. Med. VIII 1,3: CML I, p. 363,20sq.

1 ἐπικοινότερον V αἰεί *om.* V 2 σηραγγῶδές] σειραιτῶδες V ἐστιν *om.* B 5 ὑγρὰ και πολλὰ B εἰ] ἡ B 6 ἔνι δ' V: ἔνεστιν B: *corr. Kühlewein* 7 σκληρότητι ... μαλθακότητι ... κοιλότητι Ho[2] νῦν B V: οὖν *Corn., Portus* 11 ἑαυτῶ V ταυτης B 12 υπεστην B δὴ ὅτι] διότ V: διότι *recc.* 14 τρωθεις *in* τρωθεισων *mut.* B[2] 15 φλᾶταί τε] φλατεται B 16 ἐστι *post* χαλεπώτερα *trsp.* B 17 ἐξ ἴσων *Erm.* *lacunam indicavi;* καὶ ἐλασσόνων *addiderim*: καὶ ἡσσόνων *add. Littré* 18 ἀποθνήσκειν V ὁ *om.* V 22 υπο λεπτω τε γαρ B: ὑπολεπτώτεταος V: *corr.* Ho[2] ταύτην B V: *corr.* B[3] 23 ὀλίγη V 25 ἐστὶν V 28 τὸ[1] – ὄπισθεν] τοῦ ὀστέου πᾶν τὸ ὀστέον V 29 πᾶν V 30 τοῦτο] ταύτῃ *Reinh.* 31 ἐόντων *coni. Littré*: ἁπάντων B V ὁμοίως B *post* μεζόνων *add.* η B 32 μιονος B, *in* μειόνων *mut.* B[3]: μειόνων V: *del. Littré* τιτρωσκόμενος *in* -μένων *mut.* B[3] 33 ἔσω *om.* V καὶ ἣν V ἄνθρωπος V

more porous bone and into the diploe. And the diploe is the most porous and
the softest part, especially full of empty spaces. Indeed, the entire skull, ex- 6
cept a very small part, the outermost and innermost layers, is like a sponge,
and the bone contains within it many moist fleshy areas of similar appear-
ance, and, if one rubs them with the fingers, blood will come from them.
There are also in the bone rather thin hollow vessels full of blood. This, then,
is the situation regarding hardness, softness and porosity.

2. But, in respect to thickness and thinness, the bone at the bregma is
the thinnest and weakest of the entire skull, and in this part of the skull the
bone has the least and thinnest flesh over it, and there is the most brain under
this part of the skull. The result of such an arrangement is that, when some- 2
one is wounded equally or less – the wounds and weapons being the same
size or smaller – the bone in this part of the skull is more readily crushed,
fractured or crushed in, and (the injuries) are more often fatal, and medical
cure and escape from death more difficult (with wounds) here than in any
other part of the head. When equal +or smaller+[1] wounds are sustained, the
person who is wounded the same or less and who is going, in any case, to die
from the wound, dies within a shorter time when he has the wound in this
part of the skull rather than anywhere else. For at the bregma the brain is 3
most rapidly and acutely sensitive to the ills that occur in the flesh and the
bone, since at this spot the brain is under the thinnest bone and the least
flesh, and the greatest mass of the brain lies under the bregma. Of the other 4
parts, that at the temples is weakest. For at the temple is the junction of the
lower jaw with the cranium and here there is up and down movement, as of a
joint. Also near it is the organ of hearing, and through the temple stretches a
hollow and powerful blood vessel.

All of the skull behind the vertex and the ears is stronger than any part 5
in front, and this bone has a larger and deeper layer of flesh over it. The re- 6
sult of these conditions is that, when someone is wounded to the same degree
or more severely, with injuries and weapons that are alike and equal or
greater, in this part of the head the bone is less seriously fractured and
crushed in. And if a person is going to die in any case from the wound, he

1 +or smaller+: see the app. crit.

ἄλλως ἐκ τοῦ τρώματος, ὁ ἐν τῷ ὄπισθεν τῆς κεφαλῆς ἔχων τὸ τρῶμα ἐν
πλείονι χρόνῳ ἀποθανεῖται. ἐν πλείονι γὰρ χρόνῳ τὸ ὀστέον ἐμπυΐσκε-
5 ταί / τε καὶ διαπυΐσκεται κάτω ἐπὶ τὸν ἐγκέφαλον διὰ τὴν παχύτητα τοῦ
ὀστέου. καὶ ἐλάσσων ταύτῃ τῆς κεφαλῆς ὁ ἐγκέφαλος ὕπεστι. καὶ πλέονες
ἐκφυγγάνουσι τὸν θάνατον τῶν ὄπισθεν τιτρωσκομένων τῆς κεφαλῆς ὡς
ἐπὶ τὸ πολὺ ἢ τῶν ἔμπροσθεν. καὶ ἐν χειμῶνι πλείονα χρόνον ζῇ ὤνθρωπος
ἢ ἐν θέρει, ὅστις ἂν καὶ ἄλλως μέλλῃ ἀποθανεῖσθαι ἐκ τοῦ τρώματος,
ὅπου ἂν τῆς κεφαλῆς ἔχῃ τὸ τρῶμα.
194 3. Αἱ δὲ ἕδραι τῶν βελέων τῶν ὀξέων καὶ κουφοτέρων, αὐ|ταὶ ἐπὶ σφέ-
ων αὐτέων γινόμεναι ἐν τῷ ὀστέῳ ἄνευ ῥωγμῆς τε καὶ φλάσιος καὶ ἔσω ἐσ-
φλάσιος – αὗται δὲ γίνονται ὁμοίως ἔν τε τῷ ἔμπροσθεν τῆς κεφαλῆς καὶ
τῷ ὄπισθεν –, ἐκ τουτέων ὁ θάνατος οὐ γίνεται κατά γε δίκην, οὐδ' ἢν γέ-
2 νηται. ῥαφὴ δὲ ἐν ἕλκει φανεῖσα ὀστέου ψιλωθέντος, πανταχοῦ τῆς κεφα-
λῆς τοῦ ἕλκεος γενομένου, ἀσθενέστατον γίνεται τῇ τρώσει καὶ τῷ βέλει
ἀντέχειν, εἰ τύχοι τὸ βέλος ἐς αὐτὴν τὴν ῥαφὴν στηριχθέν. πάντων δὲ μά-
λιστα, ἢν τὸ ἕλκος ἐν τῷ βρέγματι γενόμενον κατὰ τὸ ἀσθενέστατον τῆς
κεφαλῆς, καὶ αἱ ῥαφαὶ εἰ τύχοιεν ἐοῦσαι [ἢ] περὶ τὸ ἕλκος καὶ τὸ βέλος αὐ-
τέων τύχοι τῶν ῥαφέων. /
6 4. Τιτρώσκεται δὲ ὀστέον τὸ ἐν τῇ κεφαλῇ τοσούσδε τρόπους, τῶν δὲ
196 τρόπων ἑκάστου πλείονες ἰδέαι γίνονται τοῦ κατήγματος | ἐν τῇ τρώσει.
2 ὀστέον ῥήγνυται τιτρωσκόμενον καὶ τῇ ῥωγμῇ ἐν τῷ περιέχοντι ὀστέῳ
τὴν ῥωγμὴν ἀνάγκη φλάσιν προσγενέσθαι, ἥνπερ ῥαγῇ. τῶν γὰρ βελέων ὅ
τι περ ῥήγνυσι τὸ ὀστέον, τὸ αὐτὸ τοῦτο καὶ φλᾷ τὸ ὀστέον ἢ μᾶλλον ἢ
ἧσσον, αὐτό τε, ἐν ᾧπερ καὶ ῥήγνυσι τὴν ῥωγμήν, καὶ τὰ περιέχοντα
3 ὀστέα τὴν ῥωγμήν. εἷς οὗτος τρόπος. ' ἰδέαι δὲ ῥωγμέων παντοῖαι γίνον-
ται. καὶ γὰρ λεπτότεραί τε καὶ λεπταὶ πάνυ, ὥστε οὐ καταφανεῖς γίνον-
ται, ἔστιν αἳ τῶν ῥωγμέων, οὔτε αὐτίκα μετὰ τὴν τρῶσιν οὐδὲ ἐν τῇσιν

6–8] *cf.* Hipp. De ulc. 5: VI 404,21sq. L. 9 Αἱ – ὀξέων] schol. *in* Orib. Coll. med. rel. XLVI 21,1: CMG VI 2,1, p. 227,25 ἕδραι] *cf.* Gal. *ap.* Orib. Coll. med. rel. XLVI 21,1: CMG VI 2,1, p. 227,27–29 τῶν^{I} – κουφοτέρων] *cf.* Gal. *ap.* Orib. Coll. med. rel. XLVI 21,1: CMG VI 2,1, p. 227,29–31 10 ῥωγμῆς] *cf.* Paul. Aeg. VI 90,1: CMG IX 2, p. 136,9sq. φλάσιος] *cf.* Sor. De signis fract. 9: CMG IV, p. 156,14–16 Paul. Aeg. VI 90,2: CMG IX 2, p. 137,1–9 ἐσφλάσιος] *cf.* Gal. *ap.* Orib. Coll. med. rel. XLVI 21,1. 10: CMG VI 2,1, p. 227,32–35; 228,29–31 19 Τιτρώσκεται – τρόπους] *cit.* Gal. In Hipp. De off. med. comm. I 6: XVIII B 672,11sq. K. 21 τῇ – 22] *cf.* Gal. *ap.* Orib. Coll. med. rel. XLVI 21,10: CMG VI 2,1, p. 228,26–28

1 αλλος B ὁ *om.* V ἐν τῷ] εκ τοῦ B 1sq. ἐν^{II} – ἀποθανεῖται *om.* B, *in marg. add.* B^{2} 4 ελασσω ταυτης B υπεστη B 6 ἄνθρωπος V 7 *ante* ὅστις *add.* ἡ B ἂν *om.* V μέλλει V 8 ἂν] οὖν V ἔχει B: ἔχων V: *corr. Kühlewein* 9 αὐταὶ *scr. Littré*: αυται B: αὗταὶ V 10 ἄνευ ῥωγμῆς] τὰ νεῦρα ἀγμῆς V 11 δ' ἐπιγίνονται B 12 *ante* τῷ *add.* ἐν V ἐκ τουτέων] εξ ων B θάνανατος V 15 εωυτην B 16 ἢν τὸ ἕλκος *coni. Erm.*: ἢν τὸ βέλος B V: *del. Scal.* 17 ἢ *om. Ald.*: *seclusi* 19 τῇ *om.* V: *hab. Gal.* τοσούσδε] κατὰ τόσους *Gal.* 21 τῇ – ἐν *om.* V τῆς ῥώγμης B: *corr. Kühlewein* 22 προσγιγνεσθαι B ᾗπερ ἂν *Erm.* 23 τερ B 24sq. καὶ^{II} – ῥωγμήν *om.* V 26 λεπταὶ] λεπτοταται B ὥστε οὐ] ὀστέου V 27 ἐστι δε των B, *in* ἐστί δ' αἴτιον *(?) mut.* B^{2}: ἔστι δ' αἴτιον V: ἐστι δ' αἳ τῶν N: *corr. Littré*: ἔνιαι τῶν *Foes. in adn.* οὐδὲ] οὔτ' V

who has his wound at the back of the head will take a longer time to die. For suppuration of the bone takes a longer time to occur and to penetrate down to the brain because of the thickness of the bone. Also less brain lies under this part of the skull. And, generally, more of those wounded in the back of the head escape death than (of those wounded) in the front. Also, whoever is going in any case to die from his wound, wherever on the head he may have the wound, lives longer in winter than in summer.

3. *Hedrai* of sharp, light weapons, when they occur by themselves in the
bone, without fracture, crush-injury or depressed crush-injury (depressed
fracture) – and they occur equally in the front and the back of the head –,
do not, at least as a natural consequence, cause death, even if it happens. But 2
a suture, appearing in a wound when the bone has been laid bare, wherever
in the skull the wound may be, is the weakest spot to withstand injury or
weapon if the weapon happens to lodge in the suture itself. This is especially
so if the wound occurs in the bregma, at the weakest spot in the skull, and if
the sutures happen to be near the wound and the weapon strikes the sutures
themselves.

4. Skull injuries are of a number of types, and for each type several
forms of injury occur in the wounding. The skull is fractured when injured 2
and, in addition to the fracture, a crush-injury necessarily occurs in the bone
surrounding the fracture, if (the skull) is indeed fractured. For the very weap-
on that fractures the skull also crushes it to a greater or lesser extent, both at
the fracture site and also in the bones surrounding the fracture. This is one
type. | The forms of fractures are manifold. For some fractures are rather thin 3
and very thin so as not to be evident, either immediately after the injury or in

200 ἡμέρῃσιν, ἐν ᾗσιν ἂν καὶ πόνων ὄφελος γένοιτο ⟨καὶ⟩ | τοῦ θανάτου τῷ ἀν-
θρώπῳ. αἱ δ' αὖ παχύτεραί τε καὶ εὐρύτεραι ῥήγνυνται τῶν ῥωγμέων, ἔνι-
4 αι δὲ καὶ πάνυ εὐρεῖαι. ἔστι δὲ αὐτέων καὶ αἳ μὲν ἐπὶ μακρότερον ῥήγνυν-
ται, αἳ δ' ἐπὶ βραχύτερον, καὶ αἱ μὲν ἰθύτεραι, αἱ δὲ ἰθεῖαι πάνυ, αἱ δὲ καμ-
7 πυλώτεραί τε καὶ ⟨πάνυ⟩ καμπύλαι, καὶ ⟨αἱ μὲν⟩ / βαθύτεραι, αἱ δὲ ἐς τὸ
κάτω καὶ διὰ παντὸς τοῦ ὀστέου.

5. Φλασθείη δ' ἂν τὸ ὀστέον μένον ἐν τῇ ἑωυτοῦ φύσει, καὶ ῥωγμὴ τῇ
φλάσει οὐκ ἂν προσγένοιτο ἐν τῷ ὀστέῳ οὐδεμία. δεύτερος οὗτος τρόπος.
2 ἰδέαι δὲ τῆς φλάσιος πλείους γίνονται· καὶ γὰρ μᾶλλόν τε καὶ ἧσσον φλᾶ-
ται καὶ ἐς βαθύτερόν τε καὶ διὰ παντὸς τοῦ ὀστέου καὶ ἧσσον ἐς βαθὺ καὶ
οὐ διὰ παντὸς τοῦ ὀστέου καὶ ἐπὶ πλέον τε καὶ ἔλασσον μήκεός τε καὶ
3 πλατύτητος. ἀλλὰ οὐ τουτέων τῶν ἰδεῶν οὐδεμίαν ἔστιν ἰδόντα τοῖσιν
202 ὀφθαλμοῖσι γνῶναι, ὁποίη τίς ἐστι τὴν ἰδέην καὶ ὁπόση | τις τὸ μέγεθος.
οὐδὲ γὰρ εἰ πέφλασται ἢ μὴ πέφλασται, ἐόντων πεφλασμένων καὶ τοῦ κα-
κοῦ γεγενημένου, γίνεται τοῖσιν ὀφθαλμοῖσι καταφανὲς ἰδεῖν αὐτίκα μετὰ
τὴν τρῶσιν, ὥσπερ οὐδὲ τῶν ῥωγμέων ἔνιαι ἑκὰς ἐοῦσαί τε καὶ ἐρρωγότος
τοῦ ὀστέου.

204 6. Ἐσφλᾶται τὸ ὀστέον ἐκ τῆς | φύσιος τῆς ἑωυτοῦ ἔσω σὺν ῥωγμῇ-
σιν· ἄλλως γὰρ οὐκ ἂν ἐσφλασθείη. τὸ γὰρ ἐσφλώμενον ἔσω, ἀπορρηγνύ-
8 μενόν τε καὶ καταγνύμε/νον, ἐσφλᾶται ἔσω ἀπὸ τοῦ ἄλλου ὀστέου μένον-
τος ἐν τῇ φύσει τῇ ἑωυτοῦ. καὶ δὴ οὕτω ῥωγμὴ ἂν προσείη τῇ ἐσφλάσει.
2 τρίτος οὗτος τρόπος. ¹ ἐσφλᾶται δὲ τὸ ὀστέον πολλὰς ἰδέας· καὶ γὰρ ἐπὶ
πλέον τοῦ ὀστέου καὶ ἐπ' ἔλασσον, καὶ μᾶλλόν τε καὶ ἐς βαθύτερον, καὶ
ἧσσόν τε καὶ ἐπιπολαιότερον.

7. Καὶ ἕδρης ἐγγενομένης ἐν τῷ ὀστέῳ βέλεος προσγένοιτ' ἂν ῥωγμὴ
206 τῇ ἕδρῃ. τῇ τε ῥωγμῇ καὶ φλάσιν προσγενέσθαι ἀναγκαῖόν ἐστιν ἢ | μᾶλ-
λον ἢ ἧσσον, ἥνπερ καὶ ῥωγμὴ προσγένηται, ἔνθαπερ καὶ ἕδρη ἐγένετο καὶ
ἡ ῥωγμὴ ⟨καὶ⟩ ἐν τῷ ὀστέῳ τῷ περιέχοντι τήν τε ἕδρην καὶ τὴν ῥωγμήν.

7–8 τρόπος] *cit.* Gal. In Hipp. De off. med. comm. I 6: XVIII B 672,14–16 K. 18 Ἐσφλᾶται – ῥωγμῇσιν] *cf.* Gal. *ap.* Orib. Coll. med. rel. XLVI 21,10: CMG VI 2,1, p. 228, 29sq. 22 τρίτος – τρόπος] *cit.* Gal. In Hipp. De off. med. comm. I 6: XVIII B 672,17 K. 25 Καὶ – βέλεος] schol. *in* Orib. Coll. med. rel. XLVI 21,10: CMG VI 2,1, p. 228,26

1 ᾗσιν] ὅσησιν B πόνων] ποιεων B καὶ^II *add. Littré, vol. X, p. XXIII* 2 αὖ] αυτεων B ῥήγνυνται] γίνονται V 3 ἔστι δὲ αὐτέων *om.* V 4 *ante* πάνυ *add.* τὲ καὶ V 5 πάνυ *add. Erm.* καὶ αἱ μὲν *scripsi*: καὶ B V: αἱ μὲν *Mart.* αἱ^II – τὸ] τε εκ του B: τε καὶ πάνυ βαθεῖαι ἐς τὸ *Mart.* 6 *post* ὀστέου *add.* καὶ (αἱ δὲ *Erm.*) ἧσσον βαθεῖαι ἐς τὸ κάτω, καὶ οὐ διὰ παντὸς τοῦ ὀστέου *Littré, Erm.* 7 Φλασθείη – μένον] θλασθείη δ' αὐτὸ ὀστέον μόνον *Gal.* τὸ *om.* B μένον *om.* V 8 ἐν *om.* V 11 οὐ *om.* V 12 οὐ *om.* V ἰδόντι V 13 ἐστι τὴν ἰδέην] ἐστιν· ἡ δὲ B ἴδην V: *corr. Ald.* τις *om.* V 14 ἢ μὴ πέφλασται *om.* V ἐον τε B, *in* ἐὸν τῶν (τῶν *in marg.*) τε *mut.* B2 16 εαιουσαι B τε *om.* Ho 19 ἔσω *om.* V 21 φλάσει B 22 ἔσφλασται V 23 *post* βαθύτερον *add.* κάτω V *post* καὶ^IV *add.* το B 25 *ante* ἐγγενομένης *add.* ἂν B γενομένης V 26 ἑδραιηι B: ἑδρέῃ V: *corr. Lind.* τῇ τε ῥωγμῇ *om.* B προσγιγνεσθαι B 27 ἥνπερ] ἧνπερ B: ἢ ἧπερ V καὶ^II] ἡ *Littré* 28 καὶ^I *add. Littré coll. p. 66,24* ῥωγμήν] φλάσιν V

the days during which the patient could be helped in his suffering and saved
from death. On the other hand, some of the fractures are rather large and
wide, and some are very wide. There are also some of them that are fractured 4
for a longer distance, others shorter, and some are fairly straight, some very
straight, and others rather curved and still others very curved; and some are
moderately deep while others extend deep and through the whole bone.

5. The bone may be crushed but retain its normal position and have no
fracture associated with the crush-injury. This is a second type. | There are 2
many forms of crush-injury: For (the bone) is crushed more or less, both to
greater depth and through the whole bone, or to less depth and not through
the whole bone, and to a greater or less extent in length and breadth. Howev- 3
er, not for a single one of these forms is it possible to discern, simply by look-
ing, what its shape is or what its extent is. For it is not evident to the eye im-
mediately after the injury whether a crush-injury has occurred or not, even
when (the bone) has been crushed and the damage done, just as some frac-
tures cannot be seen when they are far (from the site of injury) and when the
bone has been broken.

6. The bone is crushed in from its normal position, depressed with frac-
tures; for otherwise it could not be crushed in. For the crushed-in bone, both
broken off and shattered, is crushed in, depressed away from the rest of the
bone which retains its normal position. And, of course, in this situation frac-
ture will accompany the depressed crush-injury. This is a third type. | And de- 2
pressed crush-injuries have many forms; for they may extend over more or
less of the bone, may be more depressed and deeper or less depressed and
more superficial.

7. Next, when a weapon *hedrē* occurs in the skull, fracture may occur in addition to the *hedrē*. And, if fracture does in fact occur, crush-injury too, in addition to the fracture, necessarily also occurs to greater or less extent, where the *hedrē* and fracture occur and in the bone surrounding the *hedrē*

2 τέταρτος οὗτος τρόπος. | καὶ ἕδρη μὲν ἂν γένοιτο φλάσιν ἔχουσα τοῦ
208 ὀστέου περὶ αὐτήν, ῥωγμὴ δὲ οὐκ ἂν προσγένοιτο | τῇ ἕδρῃ καὶ τῇ φλάσει
9 3 ὑπὸ τοῦ βέλεος. πέμπτος οὗτος τρό/πος. | καὶ ἕδρη δὲ τοῦ βέλεος γίνεται
ἐν τῷ ὀστέῳ· ἕδρη γὰρ καλεῖται, ὅταν μένον τὸ ὀστέον ἐν τῇ ἑωυτοῦ φύσει
τὸ βέλος στηρίξαν ἐς τὸ ὀστέον δῆλον ποιήσῃ, ὅπου ἐστήριξεν. ⟨ἕκτος οὗ-
4 τος τρόπος.⟩ ἐν δὲ τῷ τρόπῳ ἑκάστῳ πλείονες ἰδέαι γίνονται· καὶ περὶ
μὲν φλάσιός τε καὶ ῥωγμῆς, κἢν ἄμφω ταῦτα προσγένηται τῇ ἕδρῃ καὶ ἢν
φλάσις μούνη γένηται, ἤδη πέφρασται, ὅτι πολλαὶ ἰδέαι γίνονται καὶ τῆς
φλάσιος καὶ τῆς ῥωγμῆς. ἡ δὲ ἕδρη αὐτὴ ἐφ' ἑωυτῆς γίνεται, μακροτέρη καὶ
βραχυτέρη ἐοῦσα καὶ καμπυλωτέρη καὶ ἰθυτέρη καὶ κυκλοτερής. καὶ πολ-
λαὶ ἄλλαι ἰδέαι τοιούτου τρόπου, ὁποῖον ἄν τι καὶ τὸ στόμα τοῦ βέλεος
ᾖ· αἱ δ' αὐταὶ καὶ βαθύτεραι τὸ κάτω καὶ μᾶλλον καὶ ἧσσον, καὶ στενότε-
ραί τε καὶ ἧσσον στεναὶ καὶ εὐρύτεραί τε καὶ πάνυ εὐρεῖαι, ᾗ διακεκόφα-
5 ται. διακοπὴ δέ, ὁποσητισοῦν γινομένη μήκεός τε καὶ εὐρύτητος ἐν τῷ
210 ὀστέῳ, ἕδρη ἐστίν, ἢν τὰ ἄλλα | ὀστέα τὰ περιέχοντα τὴν διακοπὴν μένῃ ἐν
τῇ φύσει τῇ ἑωυτῶν καὶ μὴ συνεσφλᾶται τῇ διακοπῇ ἔσω ἐκ τῆς φύσιος
τῆς ἑωυτῶν. οὕτω δὲ ἔσφλασις ἂν εἴη καὶ οὐκέτι ἕδρη.

8. Ὀστέον τιτρώσκεται ἄλλῃ τῆς κεφαλῆς ⟨ἢ⟩ ᾗ τὸ ἕλκος ἔχει ὥνθρω-
2 πος καὶ τὸ ὀστέον ἐψιλώθη τῆς σαρκός. ἕβδομος οὗτος τρόπος. | καὶ ταύ-
10 την τὴν συμφορήν, ὅταν γένηται, οὐκ ἂν ἔχοις ὠφελῆσαι οὐδέν. / οὐδὲ γάρ,
εἰ πέπονθε τὸ κακὸν τοῦτο, οὐκ ἔστιν, ὅπως χρὴ αὐτὸν ἐξελέγξαντα εἰδέ-
ναι, εἰ πέπονθε τὸ κακὸν τοῦτο ὥνθρωπος, οὐδὲ ὅπῃ τῆς κεφαλῆς.

9. Τούτων τῶν τρόπων τῆς κατήξιος ἐς πρῖσιν ἀφήκει ἥ τε φλάσις ἡ
ἀφανὴς ἰδεῖν καὶ ἤν πως τύχῃ φανερὴ γενομένη, καὶ ἡ ῥωγμὴ ἡ ἀφανὴς ἰδεῖν
καὶ ἢν φανερὴ ᾖ. καὶ ἢν ἕδρης γενομένης τοῦ βέλεος ἐν τῷ ὀστέῳ προσγένη-
ται ῥωγμὴ καὶ φλάσις τῇ ἕδρῃ καὶ ἢν φλάσις μούνη προσγένηται ἄνευ
2 ῥωγμῆς τῇ ἕδρῃ, καὶ αὕτη ἐς πρῖσιν ἀφήκει. τὸ δὲ ἔσω ἐσφλώμενον ὀστέον

1 τέταρτος – τρόπος] *cit.* Gal. In Hipp. De off. med. comm. I 6: XVIII B 672,18 K. 2 ῥωγμὴ – φλάσει] *cf.* Gal. *ap.* Orib. Coll. med. rel. XLVI 21,10: CMG VI 2,1, p. 228,28sq. 3 πέμπτος – τρόπος] *cit.* Gal. In Hipp. De off. med. comm. I 6: XVIII B 672,18 K. 5 τὸ^{I} – ὀστέον] *cf.* Gal. *ap.* Orib. Coll. med. rel. XLVI 21,1: CMG VI 2,1, p. 227,28sq. 18 Ὀστέον – ὥνθρωπος] *cf.* Cels. Med. VIII 4,6: CML I, p. 378,20sq. Gal. *ap.* Orib. Coll. med. rel. XLVI 21,8: CMG VI 2,1, p. 228,21–24 Ὀστέον – κεφαλῆς] schol. *in* Orib. Coll. med. rel. XLVI 21,8: CMG VI 2,1, p. 228,22 23 Τούτων – κατήξιος] schol. *in* Orib. Coll. med. rel. XLVI 21,15: CMG VI 2,1, p. 229,20

1 καὶ – 3 τρόπος *om.* V 4 γὰρ] δὲ V 5 ὅπη V 5sq. ἕκτος – τρόπος. *add. Erm.* 6 ειδεας B 7 τε *om.* V κἢν] ἢν V προσγίνηται V 9 αὐτὴ *scr. Littré*: αυτη B: αὕτη V 10 βραχυτέρη] μηκροτερη B 11 *ante* τοιούτου *add.* τοῦ V στόμα] σχῆμα V 12 αἱ δ' αὐταὶ καὶ βαθύτεραι *scr. Erm.*: αἱ δ' αὗται βαθυτεραι B: καὶ δ' αὐταὶ καὶ βαθύτεραί V: αὐταὶ δὲ καὶ βαθύτεραί E τὸ] τε V 13 τε^{I} – στεναὶ *om.* V τε^{II} *om.* V 13sq. ᾗ διακεκόφαται. διακοπὴ *scr. Petrequin*: ηι διακεκοπται· διακοπη B: ἢ διακεκόφαται· διακοπὴν V: Ἢ διακέκοπται διακοπὴ *Littré* 15 ἕδρην V τἄλλ' V ἐν *om.* B 16 τῇ^{II}] τοι B η διακοπη B 18 ἀλλ' ἢ V ἢ ᾗ *coni. Mart.*: ἣν B: ᾗ V ἄνθρωπος V 19 εβδομαιος B: πέμπτος *Frob.* 22 ἄνθρωπος V ὅπῃ] όκοι B 23 αφηξει B φάσις V 24 ἡ^{I} *om.* V ἡ^{II} *om.* B: ἣν V: *corr. Littré* 25 ᾖ] ἢν V 26 μοῦνον V 27 αυτη B: αὐτὴ V: *corr.* Ho

and fracture. This is a fourth type. | And *hedrē* may also occur with crush-in- 2
jury of the bone around it, but without fracture being added to the *hedrē* and
crush-injury by the weapon. This is a fifth type. | And weapon *hedrē* occurs in 3
the bone; for (a skull injury) is called a *hedrē* when the weapon, lodging in
the bone, makes a clear imprint where it lodged, while the bone remains in
its normal position. This is a sixth type. | For each type there are many forms: 4
And concerning both crush-injury and fracture, if both of them accompany
the *hedrē*, or if crush-injury alone accompanies it, it has already been pointed
out that many forms occur, both of crush-injury and of fracture. And *hedrē*, in
and of itself, is longer or shorter and more curved or straighter or rounded.
And, of such a type, many other forms occur, depending on the sharp edge of
the weapon; these same forms may also be more or less deep and more or less
narrow and either fairly broad or very broad where they have formed a cleft.
For a cleft in the bone, however great its length and breadth, is a *hedrē* if the 5
other bone surrounding the cleft remains in its normal position and is not
crushed in, along with the cleft, out of its normal position. In that case it
would be a depressed crush-injury and no longer a *hedrē*.

8. The bone is injured in another part of the head than that in which
the patient has his wound and the bone is stripped of flesh. This is a seventh
type. | When this situation occurs you can do nothing to help. For, if the pa- 2
tient has suffered this damage, it is not possible by examining him to know if
he has suffered this damage or where in the head it is.

9. Of these types of injury, both crush-injury, that which is not apparent
and that which somehow becomes evident, and fracture, that which is not ap-
parent and that which is evident, come to trephination. Also, if, in the case of
a weapon *hedrē* occurring in the bone, fracture and crush-injury accompany
the *hedrē*, or if crush-injury alone, without fracture, accompanies the *hedrē*,
this case too comes to trephination. But of the cases in which the skull is 2

212 ἐκ τῆς φύσιος τῆς ἑωυτοῦ ὀλίγα τῶν πολλῶν πρίσιος δεῖται, | καὶ τὰ μάλι-
στα ἐσφλασθέντα καὶ μάλιστα καταρραγέντα, ταῦτα πρίσιος ἥκιστα κέ-
χρηται. οὐδὲ ἕδρη αὐτὴ ἐπὶ ἑωυτῆς γενομένη ἄτερ ῥωγμῆς καὶ φλάσιος,
οὐδὲ αὕτη πρίσιος δεῖται, οὐδ' ἢν διακοπὴ μεγάλη καὶ εὐρεῖα, οὐδ' αὕτη·
διακοπὴ γὰρ καὶ ἕδρη τωὐτόν ἐστιν.

10. Πρῶτον δὲ χρὴ τὸν τρωματίην σκοπεῖσθαι, ὅπῃ ἔχει τὸ τρῶμα
τῆς κεφαλῆς, εἴτ' ἐν τοῖσιν ἰσχυροτέροισιν εἴτ' ἐν τοῖσιν ἀσθενεστέροισιν,
καὶ τὰς τρίχας καταμανθάνειν τὰς περὶ τὸ ἕλκος, εἰ διακεκόφαται ὑπὸ τοῦ
βέλεος καὶ εἰ ἔσω ἤισαν ἐς τὸ τρῶμα· καὶ ἢν τοῦτο ᾖ, φάναι κινδυνεύειν τὸ
11 ὀστέον ψιλὸν / εἶναι τῆς σαρκὸς ⟨καὶ⟩ ἔχειν τι σίνος τὸ ὀστέον ὑπὸ τοῦ
2 βέλεος. ταῦτα μὲν οὖν χρὴ ἀπόπροσθεν σκεψάμενον λέξαι μὴ ἁπτόμενον
τοῦ ἀνθρώπου· ἁπτόμενον δὲ τοῦ ἀνθρώπου ἤδη πειρᾶσθαι εἰδέναι σάφα,
εἰ ἔστι ψιλὸν τὸ ὀστέον τῆς σαρκὸς ἢ οὔ. καὶ ἢν μὲν καταφανὲς ᾖ τὸ ὀστέ-
ον τοῖσιν ὀφθαλμοῖσι ψιλὸν ⟨ἐόν⟩ – εἰ δὲ μή, τῇ μήλῃ σκέψασθαι. καὶ ἢν
214 μὲν εὕρῃς | ψιλὸν ἐὸν τὸ ὀστέον τῆς σαρκὸς καὶ μὴ ὑγιὲς ἀπὸ τοῦ τρώμα-
τος, χρὴ τοῦ ἐν τῷ ὀστέῳ ἐόντος τὴν διάγνωσιν πρῶτα ποιεῖσθαι ὁρῶντα,
3 ὅσον τέ ἐστι τὸ κακὸν καὶ τίνος δεῖται ἔργου. χρὴ δὲ καὶ ἐρωτᾶν τὸν τε-
τρωμένον, ὅπως ἔπαθε καὶ τίνα τρόπον. ἢν δὲ μὴ καταφανὲς ᾖ τὸ ὀστέον, εἰ
ἔχει τι κακὸν ἢ μὴ ἔχει, πολλῷ ἔτι χρὴ μᾶλλον τὴν ἐρώτησιν ποιεῖσθαι ⟨ἢ⟩
ψιλοῦ γε ἐόντος τοῦ ὀστέου, τὸ τρῶμα ὅπως ἐγένετο καὶ ὅντινα τρόπον.
τὰς γὰρ φλάσιας καὶ τὰς ῥωγμὰς τὰς οὐ φαινομένας ἐν τῷ ὀστέῳ, ἐνεού-
σας δέ, ἐκ τῆς ἀποκρίσιος τοῦ τετρωμένου πρῶτον διαγινώσκειν πειρᾶ-
σθαι, εἴ τι πέπονθε τούτων τὸ ὀστέον ἢ οὐ πέπονθεν. ἔπειτα δὲ καὶ λόγῳ
καὶ ἔργῳ ἐξελέγχειν πλὴν μηλώσιος. μήλωσις γὰρ οὐκ ἐξελέγχει, εἰ πέπον-
12 θέ τι τούτων τῶν κακῶν τὸ ὀστέον / καὶ εἴ τι ἐνέχει ἐν ἑωυτῷ ἢ οὐ πέπον-
4 θεν. ἀλλ' ἕδρην τε τοῦ βέλεος ἐλέγχει μήλωσις, καὶ ἢν ἐμφλασθῇ τὸ ὀστέον
ἔσω ἐκ τῆς φύσιος τῆς ἑωυτοῦ καὶ ἢν ἰσχυρῶς ῥαγῇ τὸ ὀστέον, ἅπερ καὶ
τοῖσιν ὀφθαλμοῖσι καταφανέα ἐστὶν ὁρῶντα γινώσκειν.

11. Ῥήγνυται δὲ τὸ ὀστέον τάς τε ἀφανέας ῥωγμὰς καὶ τὰς φανεράς,

5 διακοπὴ – ἐστιν] *cf. infra*, p. 76,3sq.; 78,3sq. Gal. *ap.* Orib. Coll. med. rel. XLVI 21,1: CMG VI 2,1, p. 227,27 14 τῇ μήλῃ σκέψασθαι] *cf.* Cels. Med. VIII 4,2: CML I, p. 377,27 Heliod. *ap.* Orib. Coll. med. rel. XLVI 7,1sq.: CMG VI 2,1, p. 216,28–217,2 Paul. Aeg. VI 90,3: CMG IX 2, p. 138,2 26 ἐλέγχει μήλωσις] *cf.* Hipp. De morbis I 6: p. 16, 13sq. Wittern = VI 150,16 L.

1 προσδεῖται V 1sq. καὶ – ἐσφλασθέντα *om.* B 2 κέχρηται] δειται B 3 αὔτη V ἑωυτῆς] οιαυτης B γιγνομενη B 4 αὕτη[I] *scr. Withington*: αυτη B: αὐτὴ V ἢν διακοπὴ] ἡ διαπὴ *(sic)* ἢν V 7 εἴτ'[I] – ἰσχυροτέροισιν *om.* V 8 διακεκόφαται] καὶ διακεκομεναι εισιν B 9 εἴησαν B V: *corr. Littré* καὶ[II] – φάναι *post* σαρκὸς *(lin. 10) trsp.* V ᾖ] ην B 10 καὶ *add. Littré* τι] τοι V: τε *Reinh.* 11 ἀποπρισθεν B 12 τοῦ ἀνθρώπου[II] *om.* V 13 ἢ] ει B τὸ ὀστέον[II] *post* ὀφθαλμοῖσι *(lin. 14) trsp.* V 14 ἐόν *sec. Reinh.* (ἐὸν ψιλόν) *addidi* σκέπεσθαι (τ *suprascr.*) V 17 τέ *om.* B ἔργου] ἐρίου V 18 ᾖ] ει B 19 κακὸν] νοσημα B ἢ[I]] εἰ B ἢ[II] *add. Erm.* 20 γε ἐόντος] τεοντος B: τὲ ἐόντος V: ἐόντος *Littré*: *corr. Erm.* 21 φάσηας V 22 ὑποκρίσηος V 23 τουτ(ε)ω B V: τοῦτο *Foes.*: τουτέων *Littré*: *corr. Kühlewein*: τοιοῦτον *Corn.* 24 ἐξελέγχειν] ἐξελέγχοντα V 25 τι[I] *om.* V τούτω V ἔχει V ἑαυτῷ V 26 ἐξελέγχει V ἢν ἐμφλασθῇ] ει ενεφλασθη B 27 ισχυρος B

crushed in, out of its normal position, only a few require trephination, and those that are the most crushed-in and most severely fractured need trephination least. Nor does *hedrē,* in and of itself, without fracture and crush-injury, require trephination, not even if the cleft is large and broad; for cleft and *hedrē* are the same.

10. First it is necessary to inspect the wounded person to see where the
head wound is, whether in the stronger parts or in the weaker, and to exam-
ine closely the hair around the site of injury to see if it has been severed by
the weapon and if it went into the wound; if this is the case, state it is likely
that the bone is stripped bare of flesh and the bone has sustained some sort of
injury from the weapon. These things should be said while you observe at a 2
distance, not touching the patient; but then, touching the patient, try to make
sure if the bone is bare of flesh or not. And if the bone is bare and clearly
visible to the eyes, (well and good); but if not, examine it with the probe. And
if you find the bone bare of flesh and unsound as a result of the injury, you
must first diagnose the condition of the bone, seeing how great the dam-
age is and what sort of treatment is required. You should also ask the injured 3
person how he sustained the injury and in what manner it occurred. And if
the bone is not visible, to show if it has any damage or not, then it is much
more necessary, than when the bone is bare, to inquire how he sustained the
injury and in what manner it occurred. For, in the case of crush-injuries and
fractures that are not apparent in the bone but are there, you should try first
to discern from the patient's reply if the bone has suffered any of these or
not. And then prove your diagnosis by reasoning and by examination, short of
probing. For probing does not prove if the bone has suffered, and contains
within it, any damage of these sorts or not. Probing does, however, prove the 4
existence of a weapon *hedrē* and whether the bone is crushed in, displaced
from its normal position, and whether it is severely fractured, conditions
which are also clearly apparent to the eyes on inspection.

11. The bone is fractured, sustaining either fractures difficult to see or

καὶ φλᾶται τὰς ἀφανέας φλάσιας, καὶ ἐσφλᾶται ἔσω ἐκ τῆς φύσιος τῆς
216 ἑωυτοῦ, μᾶλλον ὅταν ἕτερος ὑφ' ἑτέρου τιτρώ|σκηται ἐπίτηδες τρῶσαι
βουλομένου ἢ ὅταν ἀέκοντος, καὶ ὅταν ἐξ ὑψηλοτέρου γίνηται ἡ βολὴ ἢ ἡ
πληγή, ὁποτέρη ἂν ᾖ, μᾶλλον ἢ ὅταν ἐξ ἰσοπέδου τοῦ χωρίου, καὶ ἢν περι-
κρατῇ τῇ χειρὶ τὸ βέλος, ἤν τε βάλλῃ ἤν τε τύπτῃ, καὶ ἰσχυρότερος ἐὼν
2 ἀσθενέστερον τιτρώσκῃ. ὅσοι δὲ πίπτοντες τιτρώσκονται πρός τε τὸ
ὀστέον καὶ αὐτὸ τὸ ὀστέον, ὁ ἀπὸ ὑψηλοτάτου πίπτων καὶ ἐπὶ σκληρό-
218 τατον καὶ ἀμβλύτατον, τούτῳ κίνδυνος τὸ | ὀστέον ῥαγῆναι καὶ φλασθῆ-
ναι καὶ ἔσω ἐσφλασθῆναι ἐκ τῆς φύσιος τῆς ἑωυτοῦ. τῷ δ' ἐξ ἰσοπέδου
13 μᾶλλον τοῦ χωρίου πί/πτοντι καὶ ἐπὶ μαλθακώτερον, ἧσσον ταῦτα πά-
3 σχει τὸ ὀστέον ἢ οὐκ ἂν πάθοι. ὅσα δ' ἐσπίπτοντα ἐς τὴν κεφαλὴν βέλεα
τιτρώσκει πρός τε τὸ ὀστέον καὶ αὐτὸ τὸ ὀστέον, τὸ ἀπὸ ὑψηλοτάτου ἐμ-
πεσὸν καὶ ἥκιστα ἐξ ἰσοπέδου, καὶ σκληρότατόν τε ἅμα καὶ ἀμβλύτατον
καὶ βαρύτατον καὶ ἥκιστα κοῦφον καὶ ἥκιστα ὀξὺ καὶ μαλθακόν, τοῦτο ἂν
4 ῥήξειε τὸ ὀστέον καὶ φλάσειε. καὶ μάλιστά γε κίνδυνος ταῦτα πάσχειν τὸ
ὀστέον, ὅταν ταῦτά τε γίνηται καὶ ἐς ἰθὺ τρωθῇ καὶ κατ' ἀντίον γένηται
τὸ ὀστέον τοῦ βέλεος, ἤν τε πληγῇ ἐκ χειρὸς ἤν τε βληθῇ ἤν τέ τι ἐμπέσῃ
αὐτῷ, καὶ ἢν αὐτὸς καταπεσὼν τρωθῇ, καὶ ὁπωσοῦν τρωθεὶς κατ' ἀντίον
5 γενομένου τοῦ ὀστέου τῷ βέλει. τὰ δ' ἐς πλάγιον τοῦ ὀστέου παρασύραν-
τα βέλεα ἧσσον καὶ ῥήγνυσι τὸ ὀστέον καὶ φλᾷ καὶ ἔσω ἐσφλᾷ, κἢν ψιλω-
θῇ τὸ ὀστέον τῆς σαρκός. ἔνια δὲ τῶν τρωμάτων τῶν οὕτω τρωθέντων οὐ-
δὲ ψιλοῦται τὸ ὀστέον τῆς σαρκός.
6 Τῶν δὲ βελέων ῥήγνυσι μάλιστα τὸ ὀστέον τάς τε φανερὰς ῥωγμὰς
220 καὶ | τὰς ἀφανέας καὶ φλᾷ τε καὶ ἐσφλᾷ ἔσω ἐκ τῆς φύσιος τῆς ἑωυτοῦ τὸ
ὀστέον τὰ στρογγύλα τε καὶ περιφερέα καὶ ἀρτίστομα, ἀμβλέα τε ἐόντα
14 καὶ / βαρέα καὶ σκληρά. καὶ τὴν σάρκα ταῦτα φλᾷ τε καὶ πέπειραν ποιεῖ
καὶ κόπτει. καὶ τὰ ἕλκεα γίνεται ὑπὸ τῶν τοιούτων βελέων ἔς τε πλάγιον
καὶ ἐν κύκλῳ ὑπόκοιλα, καὶ διάπυά τε μᾶλλον γίνεται καὶ ὑγρά ἐστι καὶ
ἐπὶ πλέονα χρόνον καθαίρεται. ἀνάγκη γὰρ τὰς σάρκας τὰς φλασθείσας

2sq. τρῶσαι – ἀέκοντος] *cf.* Hipp. De liquid. usu 6: CMG I 1, p. 90,7 13–16 ἥκιστα ἐξ ἰσοπέδου ... καὶ κατ' ἀντίον] *cf.* Hipp. Coac. praenot. 491: V 696, 9sq. L. 23–26] *cf.* Hipp. Coac. praenot. 491: V 696,8sq. L. 29sq.] *cf. infra*, p. 84,15sq. Hipp. De ulc. 1: VI 402,9–11 L.

1 ἔσω] εω B 2 μάλιστα B V: *correxi* τιτρωσκόμενος B V: *correxi* τρωσαν B 3 βουλόμενος B V: *corr. Scal.* ἀέκοντος – ὅταν^{II} *om.* V ἀέκοντος *deliberavit Littré in adn.*: ακεων B: ἀέκων *Littré* υψηλοτερους B: ὑψηλοτέρης V: *corr. Littré* γίγνεται B 4 ὁκοτερη ἡ B: ὁπότερ' ἂν ᾖ V 6 ἀσθενεστερος B: ἀσθενέστερος^{ν} N: ἀσθενεστέρως V τιτρώσκῃ] τιτρώσκει B V: *corr. Littré* 7 πίπτον B 8 *post* τούτῳ *add.* δε B *ante* καὶ^{II} *add.* τε V 9 δεξιω πεδου B 10 μᾶλλον *post* χωρίου *trsp.* B τοῦ *om.* V μαλθακοτατον B 11sq. τιτρωσκει βελεα B 12 τιτρώσκειν V πρός] ες B τε *om.* V καὶ – ὀστέον^{II} *om.* V ἐμπεσων B 13 επισκληροτατον B ἅμα *om.* V 14 *ante* ὀξὺ *add.* τε καὶ V 15 γε] τε B κίνδυνος *post* ὀστέον *(lin. 16) trsp.* V 16 γίνηται] γινεται B τρωθῇ καὶ] τρωθῆναι V ἐναντίον V 17 ἤν$^{I\ et\ II}$] ἂν B 19 γένοιτο V δ' ἐς] δὲ V 20 φλᾷ – ἐσφλᾷ] φλάσει εἴσω ἐς κεφαλήν V κἂν V 21 δὲ] γὰρ V 24 φλᾷ τε] φλεται B: φλᾶται V: *corr. Erm.* 25 ἀμβλια B 26 φλᾷ τε] φλεται B: φλᾶται V: *corr. Erm.* πέπειρον V 27 τε] τὸ V

those readily visible, and is crushed, sustaining crush-injuries difficult to see,
and also is crushed in, out of its normal shape (in the following circumstan-
ces): when a person is deliberately wounded by another who intends to wound
him, rather than when he is wounded unintentionally; when the cast or strike,
whichever it may be, is from above, rather than when it is from level ground;
and if a man has good control of the weapon with his hand, whether he cast it
or strike with it; and if a stronger man wounds a weaker. With regard to 2
those who, by falling, sustain injuries extending to the skull and involving the
skull itself, he who falls from a great height and onto something very hard
and blunt is in danger of fracturing his skull, crushing it or crushing it in, out
of its normal position. But in the case of someone who falls from more level
ground and onto something rather soft, his skull suffers these injuries less or
may not suffer them at all. With regard to missiles that fall on the head, in- 3
flicting wounds which extend to the bone and involve the bone itself, that
missile falling from the greatest height, farthest from (the victim's) level, and
one that is very hard, and, at the same time, very blunt and very heavy, i.e.,
least light, sharp, and soft, is the one that will fracture the bone and crush it.
And the bone is particularly apt to suffer these injuries when these circum- 4
stances occur and when the blow is straight and the bone is in the direct line
of the weapon, whether it is wielded by hand, or thrown, or whether some-
thing falls on the person, or he is wounded by falling down or wounded in
any way whatever, provided the bone is in the direct line of the weapon.
But those weapons which strike the bone obliquely are less apt to fracture, 5
crush, or crush in the bone, even if the bone is stripped of flesh. And in the
case of some of the wounds inflicted in this way, the bone is not even
stripped of flesh.

Those weapons that are especially apt to fracture the bone, causing ei- 6
ther readily visible fractures or those difficult to see, and also to crush it and
to crush it in, out of its normal position, are curved, round, smooth-tipped,
and, at the same time, blunt, heavy and hard. These (weapons) also crush the
flesh and macerate and pound it. And wounds from such weapons become
somewhat sunken, to one side or all around, and are also more apt to suppu-
rate, and they are moist, and take longer to become clean. For the crushed

7 καὶ κοπείσας πύος γενομένας ἐκτακῆναι. τὰ δὲ βέλεα τὰ προμήκεα ἐπὶ πο-
λὺ λεπτὰ ἐόντα καὶ ὀξέα καὶ κοῦφα τήν τε σάρκα διατάμνει μᾶλλον ἢ φλᾷ
καὶ τὸ ὀστέον ὡσαύτως. καὶ ἕδρην μὲν ἐμποιεῖ αὐτὸ καὶ διακόψαν – διακο-
πὴ γὰρ καὶ ἕδρη τωὐτόν ἐστι –, φλᾷ δὲ οὐ μάλα τὸ ὀστέον τὰ τοιαῦτα βέ-
λεα οὐδὲ ῥήγνυσιν οὐδ' ἐκ τῆς φύσιος ἔσω ἐσφλᾷ.
8 Ἀλλὰ χρὴ πρὸς τῇ ὄψει τῇ ἑωυτοῦ, ὅ τι ἄν σοι φαίνηται ἐν τῷ ὀστέῳ,
καὶ ἐρώτησιν ποιεῖσθαι πάντων τούτων – τοῦ γὰρ μᾶλλόν τε καὶ ἧσσον
τρωθέντος ταῦτά ἐστι σημεῖα –, καὶ ἢν ὁ τρωθεὶς καρωθῇ καὶ σκότος πε-
ριχυθῇ καὶ ἢν δῖνος ἔχῃ καὶ πέσῃ. |
222 12. Ὅταν δὲ τύχῃ ψιλωθὲν τὸ ὀστέον τῆς σαρκὸς ὑπὸ τοῦ βέλεος καὶ
τύχῃ κατ' αὐτὰς τὰς ῥαφὰς γενόμενον τὸ ἕλκος, χαλεπὸν γίνεται καὶ τὴν
ἕδρην τοῦ βέλεος φράσασθαι τὴν ἐν τῷ ἄλλῳ ὀστέῳ φανερὴν γενομένην,
15 εἴτ' ἔνεστιν ἐν τῷ ὀστέῳ εἴτε μὴ ἔνεστιν, / καὶ ἢν τύχῃ γενομένη ἡ ἕδρη ἐν
αὐτῇσι τῇσι ῥαφῇσιν. συγκλέπτει γὰρ αὐτὴ ἡ ῥαφὴ τρηχυτέρη ἐοῦσα
224 τοῦ | ἄλλου ὀστέου, καὶ οὐ διάδηλον, ὅ τι τε αὐτοῦ ῥαφή ἐστι καὶ ὅ τι τοῦ
2 βέλεος ἕδρη, ἢν μὴ κάρτα μεγάλη γένηται ἡ ἕδρη. προσγίνεται δὲ καὶ ῥῆξις
τῇ ἕδρῃ ὡς ἐπὶ τὸ πολὺ τῇ ἐν τῇσι ῥαφῇσι γινομένῃ, καὶ γίνεται καὶ αὐτὴ
ἡ ῥῆξις χαλεπωτέρη φράσασθαι ἐρρωγότος τοῦ ὀστέου, διὰ τοῦτο, ὅτι
κατ' αὐτὴν τὴν ῥαφὴν ἡ ῥῆξις γίνεται, ἢν ῥηγνύηται, ὡς ἐπὶ τὸ πολύ. ἕτοι-
226 μον γὰρ ταύτῃ ῥήγνυσθαι τὸ ὀστέον καὶ διαχαλᾶν διὰ τὴν ἀσθέ|νειαν τῆς
φύσιος τοῦ ὀστέου ταύτῃ καὶ διὰ τὴν ἀραιότητα καὶ δὴ ἅτε τῆς ῥαφῆς
ἑτοίμης ἐούσης ῥήγνυσθαι καὶ διαχαλᾶν. τὰ δ' ἄλλα ὀστέα τὰ περιέχοντα
3 τὴν ῥαφὴν μένει ἀρραγέα, ὅτι ἰσχυρότερά ἐστι τῆς ῥαφῆς. ἡ δὲ ῥῆξις ἡ κα-
τὰ τὴν ῥαφὴν γινομένη καὶ διαχάλασίς ἐστι τῆς ῥαφῆς καὶ φράσασθαι οὐκ
228 εὐ|μαρής, οὔτε ἀπὸ ἕδρης τοῦ βέλεος γενομένης ἐν τῇ ῥαφῇ ἐπειδὰν ῥαγῇ
καὶ διαχαλάσῃ, οὔτε ἢν φλασθέντος τοῦ ὀστέου κατὰ τὰς ῥαφὰς ῥαγῇ
16 καὶ διαχαλάσῃ. ἀλλ' ἔστι χαλεπώτε/ρον φράσασθαι τὴν ἀπὸ τῆς φλάσιος

3sq. διακοπὴ – μάλα] Erot. Voc. Hipp. collect. E 30: p. 37, 13–15 Nachmanson διακοπὴ – ἐστι] *cf. supra*, p. 72,5 *infra*, p. 78,3sq. 8 καὶ[I] – 9] *cf. infra*, p. 82,12sq. Hipp. Coac. praenot. 489: V 696,2–4 L. Prorrh. II 14: IX 38,6 L. Cels. Med. VIII 4,1: CML I, p. 377,15–19 Paul. Aeg. VI 90,3: CMG IX 2, p. 137,22sq. Hipp. Epid. V 23; VII 32: V 222,17sq.; 402,1sq. L. 9 δῖνος] Erot. Voc. Hipp. collect. Δ 11: p. 33,4–6 Nachmanson 14 συγκλέπτει ... ῥαφὴ] Erot. Voc. Hipp. collect. Σ 43: p. 80,16–18 Nachmanson 17 καὶ[I] – 19 γίνεται] *cf.* Hipp. Coac. praenot. 491: V 696,7sq. L.

1 πύον V τὰ[II]] καὶ V 2 ὀξεια B 3 καὶ[II] *om.* B αὐτὸ καὶ διακόψαντα *Erm.*: αὐτῷ καὶ διακοπὴν *Reinh.* 9 ἢν *om.* V εχει B: *corr.* N: ἢ V 12 φρασεσθαι B γινομένην V 13 ἔνεστιν ἐν] ενέστι μεν B καὶ ἢν] ἤν τε V γινομένη V 14 ῥαφιησιν B συνκλεπτη B: συμβλέπει V 15 ῥαφην B 16 *ante* ἕδρη[I] *add.* ἡ B 17 τὸ πολὺ τῇ] τόπου αυτησιν B: τὸ πουλὺ αὕτη V: *corr. Littré* γινομένῃ] γινομένησι B V: γινομένη *Ald.*: *corr. Littré* αὐτῇ V 18 φράσεσθαι B 19 ἡ *bis scr.* B 20 διὰ τὴν *om.* V 21 δὴ ἅτε] διά τε V 22 τὰ δ' ἄλλα] τ' ἄλλα τὰ V ὀστέα *post* περιέχοντα *trsp.* B 23 μένει] μὲν εἰ V *ante* ὅτι *add.* τε καὶ B ισχυροτατα B 24 διαχαλασιης B 25 οὔτε] ουτε η B: οὔτε εἰ N: ἢ οὔτε V: *correxi*: οὔτε ἢν (... ῥαγῇ καὶ διαχαλάσῃ) *Littré*: οὔτε ἢν (..., ἐπειδὰν ῥαγῇ, καὶ διαχαλάσῃ) *Kühlewein* ὑπὸ V 26 οὔτε – 27 διαχαλάσῃ *om.* V ῥαφὰς *coni. Littré*: σαρκας B 27 διαχαλασθη B: *corr. Littré*

and pounded flesh must become pus and melt away. Elongated weapons, being for the most part slender, sharp and light, cut through the flesh rather than crush it, and do the same to the bone. The weapon produces a *hedrē*, and it does this by cleaving through it – for a cleft and a *hedrē* are the same thing – but such weapons do not actually crush the bone or break it or crush it in out of its normal position. 7

So, in addition to your visual inspection of what may be seen in the bone, you must also inquire about all these matters – for these are indications of a patient's being injured to a greater or lesser extent – and (inquire) whether the patient was stunned and darkness poured over him and whether he had vertigo and fell down. 8

12. When it happens that the skull is stripped bare of flesh by the weapon and that the wound occurs in the region of the sutures themselves, it is difficult to make out the weapon *hedrē*, which would be obvious elsewhere in the skull, and (to know) whether it is present in the bone or not, especially if the *hedrē* happens to be in the sutures themselves. For the suture itself, being rougher than the rest of the bone, is deceptive, and it is not at all clear what here is suture and what is weapon *hedrē*, unless the *hedrē* is very large.
And fracture, too, commonly accompanies that *hedrē* which occurs in the sutures, and the fracture itself is more difficult to make out, even though the bone is broken, for the reason that, if there is a fracture, in most cases it occurs in the suture itself. For in this spot the skull is prone to break and come apart due to the natural weakness of the bone there and to its looseness, and especially to the fact that the suture is prone to break and come apart. But the rest of the bone, that surrounding the suture, remains unbroken because it is stronger than the suture. 2
Fracture that occurs in the suture is also a separation of the suture, and is not easy to make out, neither when the fracture and separation occur as a result of a weapon *hedrē* situated in the suture, nor if the fracture and separation occur as a result of the skull's being crushed at the site of the sutures. But fracture from crush-injury is the more difficult to 3

ῥωγμήν. συγκλέπτουσι γὰρ τὴν γνώμην καὶ τὴν ὄψιν τοῦ ἰητροῦ αὗται αἱ ῥαφαὶ ῥωγμοειδεῖς φαινόμεναι καὶ τρηχύτεραι ἐοῦσαι τοῦ ἄλλου ὀστέου, ὅτι μὴ ἰσχυρῶς διεκόπη καὶ διεχάλασεν – διακοπὴ δὲ καὶ ἕδρη τωὐτόν
4 ἐστιν. ἀλλὰ χρή, εἰ κατὰ τὰς ῥαφὰς τὸ τρῶμα γένοιτο καὶ πρός γε τὸ ὀστέον καὶ ἐς τὸ ὀστέον στηρίξειε τὸ βέλος, προσέχοντα τὸν νόον ἀνευρίσκειν, ὅ τι ἂν πεπόνθῃ τὸ ὀστέον. ἀπὸ γὰρ ἴσων τε βελέων τὸ μέγεθος καὶ ὁμοίων καὶ πολλὸν [τε] ἐλασσόνων καὶ ὁμοίως τε τρωθεὶς καὶ πολὺ ἧσσον, πολλῷ μέζον ἐκτήσατο τὸ κακὸν ἐν τῷ ὀστέῳ ὁ ἐς τὰς ῥαφὰς δεξάμενος τὸ βέλος ἢ ὁ μὴ ἐς τὰς ῥαφὰς δεξάμενος. καὶ τούτων τὰ πολλὰ πρίεσθαι δεῖ. ἀλλ' οὐ χρὴ αὐτὰς τὰς ῥαφὰς πρίειν, ἀλλ' ἀποχωρήσαντα ἐν τῷ πλησίον ὀστέῳ τὴν πρῖσιν ποιεῖσθαι, ἣν πρίῃς.

13. Περὶ δὲ ἰήσιος τρωσίων τῶν ἐν τῇ κεφαλῇ καὶ ὅπως χρὴ ἐλέγχειν τὰς πάθας τὰς ἐν τῷ ὀστέῳ γινομένας τὰς μὴ φανεράς, ὧδέ μοι δοκεῖ· ἕλκος ἐν κεφαλῇ οὐ χρὴ τέγγειν οὐδενί, οὐδὲ οἴνῳ, ἄλλως ἥκιστα· οὐδὲ κατα-
230 17 πλάσσειν οὐδὲ μοτῷ τὴν | ἴησιν ποιεῖ/σθαι, οὐδ' ἐπιδεῖν χρὴ ἕλκος ἐν κεφαλῇ, ἣν μὴ ἐν τῷ μετώπῳ ᾖ τὸ ἕλκος ἐν τῷ ψιλῷ τῶν τριχῶν ἢ περὶ τὴν ὀφρῦν καὶ τὸν ὀφθαλμόν. ἐνταῦθα δὲ γινόμενα τὰ ἕλκεα καταπλάσιος καὶ ἐπιδέσιος μᾶλλον κέχρηται ἤ που ἄλλοθι τῆς κεφαλῆς τῆς ἄλλης· περιέχει γὰρ ἡ κεφαλὴ ἡ ἄλλη τὸ μέτωπον πᾶν· ἐκ δὲ τῶν περιεχόντων τὰ ἕλκεα, καὶ ἐν ὅτῳ ἂν ᾖ τὰ ἕλκεα, φλεγμαίνει καὶ ἐπανοιδίσκεται δι' αἵματος ἐπιρ-
2 ροήν. χρὴ δὲ οὐδὲ τὰ ἐν τῷ μετώπῳ διὰ παντὸς τοῦ χρόνου καταπλάσσειν καὶ ἐπιδεῖν, ἀλλ' ἐπειδὰν παύσηται φλεγμαίνοντα καὶ τὸ οἴδημα καταστῇ, παύσασθαι καταπλάσσοντα καὶ ἐπιδέοντα. ἐν δὲ τῇ ἄλλῃ κεφαλῇ ἕλκος οὔτε μοτοῦν χρὴ οὔτε καταπλάσσειν οὔτ' ἐπιδεῖν, εἰ μὴ καὶ τομῆς δέοιτο.

232 3 Τάμνειν δὲ χρὴ τῶν ἑλκέων τῶν ἐν τῇ κεφαλῇ γινομένων | καὶ ἐν τῷ μετώπῳ, ὅπου ἂν τὸ μὲν ὀστέον ψιλὸν ᾖ τῆς σαρκὸς καὶ δοκῇ τι σίνος ἔχειν ὑπὸ τοῦ βέλεος, τὰ δὲ ἕλκεα μὴ ἱκανὰ τὸ μέγεθος τοῦ μήκεος καὶ τῆς εὐρύτητος ἐς τὴν σκέψιν τοῦ ὀστέου, εἴ τι πέπονθεν ὑπὸ τοῦ βέλεος κακὸν καὶ ὁποῖόν τι πέπονθε καὶ ὅσον μὲν ἡ σὰρξ πέφλασται καὶ τὸ ὀστέον ἔχει τι

1–2 ῥαφαὶ] *cf.* Hipp. Epid. V 27: V 226,11sq. L. 3sq. διακοπὴ – ἐστιν] *cf. supra,* p. 72,5; 76,3sq. 10sq.] *cf.* Gal. *ap.* Orib. Coll. med. rel. XLVI 21,24: CMG VI 2,1, p. 230, 8–10 10 ἀλλ'^{I} – πρίειν] schol. *in* Orib. Coll. med. rel. XLVI 21,24: CMG VI 2,1, p. 230,8 13sq. ἕλκος – οἴνῳ] *cf.* Hipp. De ulc. 1: VI 400,2 L. 14–15 κεφαλῇ] *cf.* Hipp. De ulc. 1: VI 400,4–6 L. Gal. *ap.* Orib. Coll. med. rel. XLVI 21,39: CMG VI 2,1, p. 231, 26sq. 15 οὐδ' – κεφαλῇ] schol. *in* Orib. Coll. med. rel. XLVI 21,38: CMG VI 2,1, p. 231,24 16 ἣν – ἕλκος] schol. *in* Orib. Coll. med. rel. XLVI 21,40: CMG VI 2,1, p. 232,1 26–29 ὀστέου] *cf.* Cels. Med. VIII 4,8: CML I, p. 379,4sq.

1 αυται B: αὗται V: *corr. Erm.* 2 ῥωμοειδέες V 5 καὶ – ὀστέον^{II} *om.* V ἐς τὸ ὀστέον] ἐστωστον B: *corr. Littré* τὸν] χρηστον B 6 ἂν πεπόνθῃ] πέπονθ V τε *om.* V 7 πολλων B τε^{I} *del. Littré* τε^{II} *om.* V πολὺ] πολλω B 8 ἐς *supra lin. inser.* V δεξαμενον B 9 ἢ – δεξάμενος *om.* B πρίεσθαι] περιεσθαι ται B 10 ἀποχωρίσαι τὰ V 11 πρίῃς] περιης B 12 ὡς V ἐξελέγχειν V 14 *ante* κεφαλῇ *add.* τῇ V τείνειν V ἀλλ||ωσηκιστα B: ἀλλ' ὡς ἥκιστα N: ἄλλῳ δ' ἥκιστα *D. A. Russell (per litteras)* 15 οὐδὲ πιέζειν V: οὐδὲ ἐπιδεῖν *schol. in Orib.* 16 *post* ἕλκος *add.* ἢ V 19 ἡ ἄλλη *om.* B 20 ἐπιρροῆς V 22 εαν B 26 τῇ *om.* B τῷ *om.* V 27 ὅπη V 28 ικινα B 30 ἡ μὲν V

diagnose. For the sutures themselves, appearing like fractures and being
rougher than the rest of the bone, deceive the judgement and the eyesight of
the doctor, unless the cleft and separation are marked – cleft and *hedrē* are
the same thing. However, it is necessary, if the injury occurs in the region of 4
the sutures and the weapon comes to rest on the bone or in the bone, to pay
close attention to discover what the bone has suffered. For when the weapons
are equal, similar, or much less in size, the patient who receives (the force of)
the weapon in the sutures, even when wounded to the same extent or much
less, incurs greater damage to the skull by far than he who does not receive
(the weapon's force) in the sutures. Most of these cases require trephining.
However, you must not trephine the sutures themselves, but, keeping to one
side, perform the trephination in the adjacent bone, if you do trephine.

13. Concerning treatment of head wounds and the means necessary to
diagnose bone lesions that are not apparent, this is my opinion: A head wound
should not be moistened with anything, not even wine, or, if at all, with the
least amount; nor (should a head wound) receive a poultice or be treated with
a lint dressing or be bandaged, unless the wound is on the forehead, in the
area bare of hair, or in the region of the eyebrow and eye. Wounds occurring
in these areas have a greater need of poulticing and bandaging than those
elsewhere in the head; for the rest of the head surrounds the entire forehead,
and from the surrounding areas the wounds, wherever they may be, become
inflamed and swollen through an influx of blood. But even wounds on the 2
forehead should not be treated with poultices and bandages continuously, but
when the inflammation stops and the swelling subsides, stop applying plasters
and bandaging. But in the rest of the head a wound should not be treated with
a lint dressing, or with poultices, or with bandaging, unless it also requires incision.

Wounds in the head and forehead should be incised wherever the bone 3
is bare of flesh and seems to have some damage from the weapon but the
wounds are not sufficiently long or broad for inspection of the bone, to see if
it suffered any damage from the weapon and what sort it suffered and to
what extent the flesh has been crushed and the bone injured, or, on the other

σίνος, καὶ δ' αὖτε εἰ ἀσινές τέ ἐστι τὸ ὀστέον ὑπὸ τοῦ βέλεος καὶ μηδὲν πέ-
πονθε κακόν, καὶ ἐς τὴν ἴησιν, οἵης τινὸς δεῖται τὸ ἕλκος, ἥ τε σὰρξ καὶ ἡ
18 4 πάθη τοῦ / ὀστέου. τὰ δὴ τοιαῦτα τῶν ἑλκέων τομῆς δεῖται. ¹ καὶ ὅταν τὸ
μὲν ὀστέον ψιλωθῇ τῆς σαρκός, ὑπόκοιλα δὲ ᾖ ἐς πλάγιον ἐπὶ πολύ, ἐπ-
234 ανατάμνειν τὸ κοῖλον, ὅπου μὴ | εὐμαρές ἐστι τῷ φαρμάκῳ ἀφικέσθαι,
ὁποίῳ ἄν τινι χρῇ. καὶ τὰ κυκλοτερέα τῶν ἑλκέων καὶ ὑπόκοιλα ἐπὶ πολὺ
καὶ τὰ τοιαῦτα ἐπανατάμνων τὸν κύκλον διχῇ κατὰ μῆκος, ὥσπερ πέφυκεν
ὥνθρωπος, μακρὸν ποιεῖν τὸ ἕλκος.

5 Τάμνοντι δὲ κεφαλὴν τὰ μὲν ἄλλα τῆς κεφαλῆς ἀσφάλειαν ἔχει ταμνό-
μενα· ὁ δὲ κρόταφος καὶ ἄνωθεν ἔτι τοῦ κροτάφου, κατὰ τὴν φλέβα τὴν διὰ
τοῦ κροτάφου φερομένην, τοῦτο δὲ τὸ χωρίον μὴ τάμνειν. σπασμὸς γὰρ
ἐπιλαμβάνει τὸν τμηθέντα. καὶ ἢν μὲν ἐν τῷ ἐπ' ἀριστερὰ τμηθῇ κροτάφῳ,
τὰ ἐπὶ δεξιὰ ὁ σπασμὸς ἐπιλαμβάνει, ἢν δ' ⟨ἐν τῷ⟩ ἐπὶ [τὰ] δεξιὰ τμηθῇ
κροτάφῳ, τὰ ἐπ' ἀριστερὰ ὁ σπασμὸς ἐπιλαμβάνει.

14. Ὅταν οὖν τάμνῃς ἕλκος ἐν κεφαλῇ τοῦ ὀστέου εἵνεκα τῆς σαρκὸς
ἐψιλωμένου, θέλων εἰδέναι, εἴ τι ἔχει τὸ ὀστέον κακὸν ὑπὸ τοῦ βέλεος ἢ καὶ
19 οὐκ ἔχει, τάμνειν χρὴ τὸ μέγεθος τὴν τομήν, ὅση ἂν δοκῇ / ἀποχρῆναι. τά-
μνοντα δὲ χρὴ ἀναστεῖλαι τὴν σάρκα ἀπὸ τοῦ ὀστέου, ᾗ πρὸς τῇ μήνιγγι
236 καὶ πρὸς τῷ ὀστέῳ | πέφυκεν. ἔπειτα διαμοτῶσαι πᾶν τὸ ἕλκος μοτῷ, ὅσ-
τις εὐρύτατον τὸ ἕλκος παρέξει ἐς τὴν ὑστεραίην σὺν ἐλαχίστῳ πόνῳ. μο-
τώσαντα δὲ χρὴ καταπλάσματι χρῆσθαι, ὅσον ἄν περ χρόνον καὶ τῷ μο-
τῷ, μάζῃ ἐκ λεπτῶν ἀλφίτων· ἐν ὄξει δὲ μάσσειν, ἕψειν δὲ καὶ γλίσχρην
ποιεῖν ὡς μάλιστα.

2 Τῇ δ' ὑστεραίῃ ἡμέρῃ ἐπειδὰν ἐξέλῃς τὸν μοτὸν κατιδὼν τὸ ὀστέον, ὅ
τι πέπονθεν, ἐὰν μή σοι καταφανὴς ᾖ ἡ τρῶσις, ὁποίη τίς ἐστιν ἐν τῷ
ὀστέῳ, μηδὲ διαγινώσκῃς, εἴτε τι ἔχει τὸ ὀστέον κακὸν ἐν ἑωυτῷ ἢ καὶ οὐκ
ἔχει, τὸ δὲ βέλος δοκῇ ἀφικέσθαι ἐς τὸ ὀστέον καὶ σίνασθαι, ἐπιξύειν χρὴ
τῷ ξυστῆρι κατὰ βάθος καὶ κατὰ μῆκος τοῦ ἀνθρώπου, ὡς πέφυκε, καὶ αὖ-
τις ἐπικάρσιον τὸ ὀστέον τῶν ῥηξίων εἵνεκα τῶν ἀφανέων ἰδεῖν καὶ τῆς
φλάσιος εἵνεκα τῆς ἀφανέος τῆς οὐκ ἐσφλωμένης ἔσω ἐκ τῆς φύσιος τῆς κε-
φαλῆς τοῦ ἄλλου ὀστέου. ἐξελέγχει γὰρ ἡ ξῦσις μάλα τὸ κακόν, ἢν μὴ καὶ

6–8 ὥνθρωπος] *cf.* Hipp. De ulc. 8: VI 406,10–13 L. 6 καὶ[I] – ἑλκέων] schol. *in* Orib. Coll. med. rel. XLIII 38,3: CMG VI 2,1, p. 102,1 10–14] *cf.* Hipp. Coac. praenot. 488: V 696,1sq. L. 10sq.] *cf.* Heliod. *ap.* Orib. Coll. med. rel. XLVI 8,11: CMG VI 2,1, p. 218,21–26 19 ἔπειτα – ἕλκος] schol. *in* Orib. Coll. med. rel. XLVI 21,30. 31: CMG VI 2,1, p. 230,31; 231,5

1 αυται B 2 δεῖται τινὸς τό τε V 3 δὴ] τε B ἑλκέων] ὀστεων B καὶ ὅταν *coni. Kühlewein*: και ον ἀν B: κακὸν ἂν V 4 ἀναταμνειν B 5 ὅπη V εὐμαρές ἐστι] εὐχερὲς V 6 χρῇ *scr. Littré*: χρη B: χρή V κοικλοτερᾶ (ε supra) B: κυκλώτερα V 7 ὡς V 8 ἄνθρωπος V 10 φλεβαν B 11 ἐπιφενομενην B 12 ἐν τῷ *om.* V 13 ἢν – 14 ἐπιλαμβάνει *om.* B ἐν τῷ *add. Reinh.* τὰ[II] *om. Kühlewein*: *seclusi* 15 ταμνεις B τοῦ *om.* V 16 εἴ τι ἔχει] ἐπέχει V ἧ V 17 της τομης B: *corr. Kühlewein*: τὴν τολίην V: τὴν ὠτείλην *Ald.* ὁκοσηι ην B ἄνω χρῆναι V 18 διαστειλαι B ἣ V 19 τὸ ἕλκος πᾶν V *post* ὅστις *add.* ἂν V 21 χρὴ *om.* V περ *om.* V 22 μαζης κλεπτων B *ante* ἕψειν *add.* ἢ V 27 σινεσθαι τὴν σαρκα B *ante* χρὴ *add.* τε B 29 ἐπικάρσιον] εἰ ἧ κάρσιον V 30 εσφαλωμενης B 31 μάλα τὸ κακόν] μᾶλλον V

hand, to see if the bone is uninjured by the weapon and has suffered no damage, and, with regard to treatment, to see what sort the wound requires, both for the flesh and the bony lesion. These are the sorts of wounds that require incision. When the bone is laid bare of flesh and there is marked undermin- 4
ing to one side, open up the undermined area by incision wherever it is not easy for the medicine, whichever you use, to reach. In the case of wounds which are circular and markedly undermined, open up such wounds by incising the circumference in two places lengthwise, as the person has grown, so making the wound a long one.

If one makes an incision in the head, the other parts of the head may be 5
incised with safety; but this part, the temple and the area above it in the region of the blood vessel which traverses the temple, should not be incised. For spasm then seizes the patient. And if the incision is made in the left temple, spasm seizes the right side (of the body), and if the incision is made in the right temple, spasm seizes the left side (of the body).

14. Therefore, when you incise a head wound because the bone is stripped bare of flesh and you wish to know if the bone has, or has not, sustained any damage from the weapon, you must make the incision of a size that seems sufficient. And, as you incise, you must lift the scalp away from the bone where it adheres to the membrane (pericranium) and the bone. Then pack the entire wound with lint dressing in order to keep the wound as wide as possible until the next day with the least pain. After packing (the wound) you must use as a poultice, for as long a time as the packing, a dough made of fine barley meal; knead it with vinegar and boil it and make it as glutinous as possible.

The next day, when you take out the packing and look to see what the 2
bone has suffered, if the type of bony injury is not apparent to you, and you cannot determine if the bone has anything wrong with it or not, but the weapon appears to have reached the bone and to have injured it, you should scrape down into the bone with a rasp, both longitudinally, as regards the growth of the patient, and transversely as well, in an effort to see fractures which are not apparent and any crush-injury which is not apparent because (the injured bone) is not crushed in, away from the normal position of the rest of the skull. For rasping effectively demonstrates the damage, if these le-

238 3 ἄλλως καταφανεῖς ἔωσιν αὗται αἱ πάθαι ἐοῦσαι ἐν | τῷ ὀστέῳ. καὶ ἢν
ἕδρην ἴδῃς ἐν τῷ ὀστέῳ τοῦ βέλεος, ἐπιξύειν χρὴ αὐτήν τε τὴν ἕδρην καὶ
20 τὰ / περιέχοντα αὐτὴν ὀστέα, μὴ πολλάκις τῇ ἕδρῃ προσγένηται ῥῆξις καὶ
φλάσις, ἢ μούνη φλάσις, ἔπειτα λανθάνῃ οὐ καταφανέα ἐόντα.
4 Ἐπειδὰν δὲ ξύσῃς τὸ ὀστέον τῷ ξυστῆρι, ἢν μὲν δοκῇ ἐς πρῖσιν ἀφή-
κειν ἡ τρῶσις τοῦ ὀστέου, πρίειν χρὴ καὶ τὰς τρεῖς ἡμέρας μὴ ὑπερβάλλειν
ἀπρίωτον, ἀλλ' ἐν ταύτῃσι πρίειν ἄλλως τε καὶ τῆς θερμῆς ὥρης, ἢν ἐξ ἀρ-
5 χῆς λαμβάνῃς τὸ ἴημα. ἢν δὲ ὑποπτεύῃς μὲν τὸ ὀστέον ἐρρωγέναι ἢ πεφλά-
σθαι ἢ ἀμφότερα ταῦτα, τεκμαιρόμενος, ὅτι ἰσχυρῶς τέτρωται, ἐκ τῶν λό-
γων τοῦ τρωματίου, καὶ ὅτι ὑπὸ ἰσχυροτέρου τοῦ τρώσαντος, ἢν ἕτερος
ὑφ' ἑτέρου τρωθῇ, καὶ τὸ βέλος, ὅτῳ ἐτρώθη, ὅτι τῶν κακούργων βελέων
ἦν, ἔπειτα τὸν ἄνθρωπον ὅτι δῖνός τε ἔλαβε καὶ σκότος καὶ ἐκαρώθη καὶ
κατέπεσεν, τούτων δὲ οὕτω γινομένων, ἢν μὴ διαγινώσκῃς, εἰ ἔρρωγε τὸ
240 ὀστέον ἢ πέφλασται ἢ καὶ ἀμφότερα ταῦτα, μήτε ἄλλως ὁρῶν, δεῖ δὴ | ἐπὶ
τὸ ὀστέον τὸ τηκτὸν τὸ μελάντατον δεύσαντα τῷ μέλανι φαρμάκῳ τῷ τη-
κομένῳ στεῖλαι τὸ ἕλκος· ὑποτείνας ὀθόνιον ἐλαίῳ τέγξας, εἶτα καταπλά-
21 6 σας / τῇ μάζῃ ἐπιδῆσαι. τῇ δὲ ὑστεραίῃ ἀπολύσας, ἐκκαθήρας τὸ ἕλκος
ἐπιξῦσαι. καὶ ἢν μὴ ὑγιὲς ᾖ, ἀλλ' ἐρρώγῃ καὶ πεφλασμένον ᾖ, τὸ μὲν ἄλλο
ἔσται ὀστέον λευκὸν ἐπιξυόμενον, ἡ δὲ ῥωγμὴ καὶ ἡ φλάσις κατατακέντος
242 τοῦ | φαρμάκου δεξαμένη τὸ φάρμακον ἐς ἑωυτὴν μέλαν ἐὸν ἔσται μέλαινα
7 ἐν λευκῷ τῷ ὀστέῳ τῷ ἄλλῳ. ἀλλὰ χρὴ αὖτις τὴν ῥωγμὴν ταύτην φανεῖ-
σαν μέλαιναν ἐπιξεῖν κατὰ βάθο[υ]ς· καὶ ἢν μὲν ἐπιξύων τὴν ῥωγμὴν ἐξέλῃς
καὶ ἀφανέα ποιήσῃς, φλάσις μὲν γεγένηται τοῦ ὀστέου ἢ μᾶλλον ἢ ἧσσον,
ἥτις περ ἔρρηξε καὶ τὴν ῥωγμὴν τὴν ἀφανισθεῖσαν ὑπὸ τοῦ ξυστῆρος· ἧσ-
σον δὲ φοβερὸν καὶ ἧσσον ἂν πρῆγμα ἀπ' αὐτῆς γίνοιτο ἀφανισθείσης τῆς
8 ῥωγμῆς. ἢν δὲ κατὰ βάθο[υ]ς ᾖ καὶ μὴ ἐθέλῃ ἐξιέναι ἐπιξυομένη, ἐς πρῖσιν

6 πρίειν – 8] *cf.* Gal. *ap.* Orib. Coll. med. rel. XLVI 21,30–32: CMG VI 2,1, p. 231,1–12   7 ἄλλως – ὥρης] schol. *in* Orib. Coll. med. rel. XLVI 21,30: CMG VI 2,1, p. 231,3   12sq. δῖνός – κατέπεσεν] *cf. supra*, p. 76,8sq.   15 μέλανι φαρμάκῳ] Gal. Ling. s. dict. exolet. Hipp. explic. M: XIX 129,6sq. K.   16 στεῖλαι] Gal. Ling. s. dict. exolet. Hipp. explic. Σ: XIX 140,10 K.   ὑποτείνας – τέγξας] *cf.* Hipp. De ulc. 11: VI 410,21 L.   19 ἡ^{I} – 22] *cf.* Cels. Med. VIII 4,6: CML I, p. 378,18–20   Paul. Aeg. VI 90,3: CMG IX 2, p. 138, 3–7

1 ἐοῦσαι] αἰουσαι B   *post* ὀστέῳ *add.* τοῦ βέλεος V   2 *post* ἕδρην^{II} *add.* τοῦ βέλεος V   3 προστένηται V   4 ἢ – φλάσις^{II} *om.* B, *in marg. infer. add.* B²   5 δοκείῃ V   ἀφίκειν V   6 καὶ τὰς *e* κατὰ *corr.* V: καὶ ου δη τας B: καὶ οὐ δεῖ τὰς N   7 ὥρης, ἢν] ὡρησιν B   8 ὑποπτεύσῃς V   10 ἰσχυροῦ V   ἑτερου B   11 καὶ – ἐτρώθη *om.* B, *in marg. add.* B²   12 ὅτι] εἰ B   *ante* ἐκαρώθη *add.* εἰ B   καὶ^{III} *om.* V   14 ἄλλως ὁρῶν] ὅλως ὁρῶν δύνῃ E: ὅλως ὁρᾶν δύνῃ *Littré*   15 τίκτον V   16 στεῖλαι *om.* V   ὑποτείνειν E: ὑποτείναντα *Littré*   *post* ὑποτείνας *addiderit* δὲ *B. Maucolin (per litteras)*   τέγξαντα E *Littré*   καταπλάσαντα E *Littré*   17 ἀπολύσαντα E *Littré*   ἐκκαθήραντα E *Littré*   18 ᾖ ὑγιὲς V   19 ξυόμενον V   20 μελα‖νεον B: μελάνεον V: *corr. Frob.*   μέλαινα] μέλαν B V: *corr. Corn., Scal.*   21 ἐν] μεν B   22 ἐπιξεῖν] ἐπιξύειν *Portus*   βάθους B V: *corr.* Ho²   *post* ῥωγμὴν *add.* ταύτην φανεῖσαν μέλαιναν V *(cf. lin. 21sq.)*   23 ἀφανεαν B   ποιησεις B   24 περιερρηξεν B   25 πρῆγμα] τα πραγματα B   γένοιτο V   26 βάθους B V: *corr. Ald.*   26sq. ἀφίκει ἐς πρίσιν V

sions, although present in the bone, are not otherwise evident. And if you see 3
a weapon *hedrē* in the bone you should rasp the *hedrē* itself and the bone sur-
rounding it to prevent the situation, which often happens, of fracture and
crush-injury, or crush-injury alone, occurring in association with *hedrē,* and
then, because they are not obvious, being overlooked.

When you scrape the bone with the rasp, if the bone injury appears to 4
require trephination, you must trephine and not exceed three days without
trephination, but trephine within that time period, especially in hot weather,
if you undertake the patient's care from the beginning. And if you suspect 5
that the bone has been fractured or has sustained a crush-injury or both these,
taking as indications the fact that, from the patient's account, he has received
a severe blow, and that the blow was administered by someone stronger, if it
is a case of one person being wounded by another, and that the weapon with
which he was wounded was of a sort to cause damage, and then that the pa-
tient experienced vertigo and darkening of vision and he was stunned and fell
down, in these circumstances, if you cannot determine whether the bone has
sustained a fracture or a crush-injury or both of these, and cannot, even in an-
other way, by inspection, then you must pour onto the bone the very black so-
lution and spread this dissolved black medication over the wound; then, after
stretching linen as an under-dressing over the wound, and wetting it with oil,
and then applying a barley-meal poultice, bandage it. The next day, after re- 6
moving (the dressing) and cleaning the wound, use the rasp. And if the bone
is not healthy, but has sustained a fracture or crush-injury, the rest of the
bone, after being rasped, will be white, but the fracture and the crush-injury,
because the medication is dissolved, will have absorbed it and, because it is
black, will be black in the otherwise white bone. You must then scrape fur- 7
ther toward the depth of this black-appearing fracture, and, if in rasping you
remove the fracture and make it invisible, then there has been a crush-injury
of the bone, more or less severe, and this caused the fracture, now obliterated
by the rasp; but it will be less a cause for fear and less a matter of concern
with the fracture obliterated. But if it goes deep and will not disappear with 8

ἀφήκει ἤδη ⟨ἡ⟩ τοιαύτη συμφορή. ἀλλὰ χρὴ πρίσαντα τὰ λοιπὰ ἰητρεύειν
τὸ ἕλκος.
15. Φυλάσσεσθαι δὲ χρή, ὅπως μή τι κακὸν ἀπολαύσῃ τὸ ὀστέον
ἀπὸ τῆς σαρκός, ἢν κακῶς ἰητρεύηται. ὀστέῳ γὰρ καὶ πεπρισμένῳ καὶ ἄλ-
λως ἀπρίστῳ, ἐψιλωμένῳ δέ, καὶ ὑγιεῖ δὲ ἐόντι καὶ ἔχοντί τι σίνος ὑπὸ τοῦ
22 βέλεος, δοκέοντι δὲ ὑγιεῖ εἶναι, κίνδυνός ἐστι / μᾶλλον ὑπόπυον γενέσθαι,
ἢν μὴ καὶ ἄλλως μέλλῃ, ἢν καὶ ἡ σὰρξ ἡ περιέχουσα τὸ ὀστέον κακῶς θερα-
πεύηται καὶ φλεγμαίνῃ τε καὶ περισφίγγηται. πυρετῶδες γὰρ γίνεται καὶ
πολλοῦ φλογμοῦ πλέον· καὶ δὴ τὸ ὀστέον ἐκ τῶν περιεχουσέων σαρκῶν ἐς
ἑωυτὸ θέρμην τε καὶ φλογμὸν καὶ ἄραδον ἐμποιεῖ καὶ σφυγμὸν καὶ ὅσα
περ ἡ σὰρξ ἴσχει κακὰ ἐν ἑωυτῇ, καὶ ἐκ τούτων οὕτως ὑπόπυον γίνεται.
2 κακὸν δὲ καὶ ὑγρήν τε εἶναι τὴν σάρκα ἐν τῷ ἕλκει καὶ μυδῶσαν καὶ ἐπὶ
πολλὸν χρόνον καθαίρεσθαι. ἀλλὰ χρὴ διάπυον μὲν ποιῆσαι τὸ ἕλκος ὡς
244 τάχιστα. οὕτως γὰρ ἂν ἥκιστα φλεγμαίνοι τὰ περιέχοντα | τὸ ἕλκος καὶ
τάχιστ' ἂν καθαρὸν εἴη· ἀνάγκη γὰρ ἔχει τὰς σάρκας τὰς κοπείσας καὶ
φλασθείσας ὑπὸ τοῦ βέλεος ὑποπύους γενομένας ἐκτακῆναι. ἐπειδὰν δὲ
καθαρθῇ, ξηρότερον χρὴ γίνεσθαι τὸ ἕλκος. οὕτως γὰρ ἂν τάχιστα ὑγιὲς
γένοιτο ξηρῆς σαρκὸς βλαστούσης καὶ μὴ ὑγρῆς, καὶ οὕτως οὐκ ἂν ὑπερ-
3 σαρκήσειε τὸ ἕλκος. ὁ δὲ αὐτὸς λόγος καὶ ὑπὲρ τῆς μήνιγγος τῆς περὶ τὸν
ἐγκέφαλον· ἢν γὰρ αὐτίκα ἐκπρίσας τὸ ὀστέον καὶ ἀφελὼν ἀπὸ τῆς μήνιγ-
γος ψιλώσῃς, αὐτὴν καθαρὴν χρὴ ποιῆσαι ὡς τάχιστα καὶ ξηρήν, ὡς μὴ
23 ἐπὶ πολὺν χρόνον ὑγρὴ ἐοῦσα / μυδᾷ τε καὶ ξαίνηται· τούτων γὰρ οὕτως
γινομένων σαπῆναι αὐτὴν κίνδυνος. |
246 16. Ὀστέον δέ, ὅ τι δεῖ ἀποστῆναι ἀπὸ τοῦ ἄλλου ὀστέου ἕλκεος ἐν
κεφαλῇ γενομένου ἕδρης τε ἐούσης τοῦ βέλεος ἐν τῷ ὀστέῳ ἢ ἄλλως ἐπὶ πο-
λὺ ψιλωθέντος τοῦ ὀστέου, ἀφίσταται ἐπὶ πολὺ ἔξαιμον γενόμενον. ἀνα-
ξηραίνεται γὰρ τὸ αἷμα ἐκ τοῦ ὀστέου ὑπό τε τοῦ χρόνου καὶ ὑπὸ φαρ-
2 μάκων τῶν πλείστων. τάχιστα δ' ἂν ἀποσταίη, εἴ τις τὸ ἕλκος ὡς τάχι-
στα καθήρας ξηραίνοι τὸ λοιπὸν τό τε ἕλκος καὶ τὸ ὀστέον, καὶ τὸ μέζον
καὶ τὸ ἧσσον. τὸ γὰρ τάχιστα ἀποξηρανθὲν καὶ ἀποστρακωθὲν τοῦτο

6 ὑπόπυον] Erot. Voc. Hipp. collect. Y 15: p. 89,7 Nachmanson: ὕπομβρον ὀστέον· ὑπόνομον καὶ κάθυγρον γεγονός Gal. Ling. s. dict. exolet. Hipp. explic. Y: XIX 149,9 K.: ὕπομβρον· ὕφυγρον, ὑπόπυον *cf.* Heliod. *ap.* Orib. Coll. med. rel. XLVI 16,1: CMG VI 2,1, p. 224,2: Τὸ λεγόμενον ὑπόπυον ὀστέον 11 ὑπόπυον] *cf. supra,* lin. 6 12 μυδῶσαν] *cf.* Hipp. De ulc. 10: VI 408,16 L. 13sq. ἀλλὰ – ἕλκος] *cf.* Hipp. De ulc. 1: VI 400, 16sq. L. 15sq.] *cf. supra,* p. 74,29sq. 21sq. ὡς – μυδᾷ] *cf.* Hipp. De locis in hom. 32: VI 324,8sq. L. 26 ἔξαιμον] *cf.* Hipp. De morbis II 24: VII 38,14 L.

1 ἤδη B: ἡ δὴ V ἡ *add. Reinh.* 5 ἀπρίστῳ *om.* V δέ, καὶ *om.* V 6 ὑπόπυον] ὑπὸ πύθη V 7 μὴ *post* ἄλλως *trsp.* V 8 φλεγμαίνῃ τε] φλεγμαίνηται V *ante* περισφίγγηται *add.* ιωμενον B 9 φλεγμου B 11 ἔχει V οὕτος B: ὧδε V 12 μαδωσαν B 15 τάχιστ' ἂν] ταχιστα B 16 γιγνομενας B 18 ὑπερσαρκίση V 19 ὑπὲρ] περι B 19sq. τω ἐγκεφαλω B 22 μηδύη V ξαίνηται] ἐξαίρηται V: ἐξερῆται *Weber ap. Kühlewein* 24 δεῖ] δὴ V ἀπὸ τοῦ] δεῖ ὅτου V *ante* ἕλκεος *add.* ἐξ B 25 ἐν τῷ ὀ(στέῳ)] *hic desinit* B 26 γινόμενον V: *corr. Erm.* 29 ξηραίνοιτο V: *corr.* N 30 ἀποστρακωθὲν] ἀπεστρακὸς, ἐν V: ἀποστρακὸς, ἐν *Frob.*: *corr. Littré* τούτω V: *corr. Erm.*

rasping, at this point such a situation calls for trephination. And after trephin-
ing it is necessary to apply the remaining treatments for healing the wound.

15. Care must be taken that the bone not contract anything harmful
from the flesh if it is improperly treated. For bone that is trephined or else
untrephined but laid bare, whether it be sound or have some weapon damage
and only appear sound, is at greater risk of suppuration, even if otherwise it
would not occur, if the flesh surrounding the bone is improperly treated and
becomes inflamed and contracts. For (the flesh) becomes feverish and full of
inflammation, and then indeed from the surrounding flesh the bone draws in-
to itself heat, inflammation, irritation and throbbing and however many harm-
ful conditions the flesh has in it, and so from these becomes purulent. It is al- 2
so bad for the flesh in the wound to be moist and to ooze and to be a long
time in becoming clean. Rather, the wound should be made to suppurate as
quickly as possible. For thus the (flesh) surrounding the wound will be the
least inflamed and (the wound) will most rapidly be clean; for the flesh that
has been lacerated and crushed by the weapon must necessarily become puru-
lent and melt away. And when the wound is cleansed, it must become drier.
For thus, with dry flesh growing and not wet, the wound will very rapidly be-
come healthy and so will not produce exuberant growth of flesh. The same 3
reasoning applies also to the membrane around the brain; for if you trephine
through the bone straightaway, and remove it from the membrane, and there-
by expose (the membrane) you must make it clean and dry as soon as possible,
so that it does not, as a result of being moist a long while, begin to ooze and
to be macerated; for in these circumstances there is a risk of its becoming pu-
trid.

16. Any bone that is sure to separate from the rest of the bone when a
wound has occurred in the head and there is a weapon *hedrē* in the bone, or
when the bone has been extensively exposed in some other fashion, generally
separates after becoming bloodless. For the blood in the bone is dried up both
by time and by most medications. And (the bone) will separate most rapidly 2
if the wound is cleaned as soon as possible and after that if both the wound
and the bone are made dry, whether (the area of bone affected be) larger or
smaller. For that bone which has been most rapidly rendered dry and has be-

μάλιστα ἀφίσταται ἀπὸ τοῦ ἄλλου ὀστέου τοῦ ἐναίμου τε καὶ ζῶντος.
αὐτὸ ⟨δ'⟩ ἔξαιμόν τε γενόμενον καὶ ξηρὸν ⟨ἐν⟩ τῷ ἐναίμῳ καὶ ζῶντι μάλα
ἀφίσταται. |

248 17. Ὅσα δὲ τῶν ὀστέων ἐσφλᾶται ἔσω ἐκ τῆς φύσιος τῆς ἑωυτῶν κα-
ταρραγέντα ἢ καὶ διακοπέντα πάνυ εὐρέα, ἀκινδυνότερα τὰ τοιαῦτα γί-
νεται, ἐπὴν ἡ μῆνιγξ ὑγιὴς ᾖ. καὶ τὰ πλέοσι ῥωγμῇσιν ἐσκαταρραγέντα
καὶ εὐρυτέρῃσιν ἔτι ἀκινδυνότερα καὶ εὐμαρέστερα ἐς τὴν ἀφαίρεσιν γίνε-
24 ται. καὶ οὐ χρὴ πρίειν τῶν τοιούτων / οὐδὲν οὐδὲ κινδυνεύειν τὰ ὀστέα
πειρώμενον ἀφαιρεῖν, πρὶν ἢ αὐτόματα ἐπανίῃ †εἰκὸς πρῶτον χαλάσαν-
250 2 τος†. ἐπανέρχεται δὲ τῆς σαρκὸς | ὑποφυομένης· ὑποφύεται δ' ἐκ τῆς δι-
πλόης τοῦ ὀστέου καὶ ἐκ τοῦ ὑγιέος, ἢν ἡ ἄνωθεν μοῖρα τοῦ ὀστέου μούνη
σφακελίσῃ. οὕτω δ' ἂν τάχιστα ἥ τε σὰρξ ὑποφύοιτο καὶ βλαστάνοι καὶ
τὰ ὀστέα ἐπανίοι, εἴ τις τὸ ἕλκος ὡς τάχιστα διάπυον ποιήσας καθαρὸν
3 ποιήσειεν. καὶ ἢν διὰ παντὸς τοῦ ὀστέου ἄμφω αἱ μοῖραι ἐσφλασθῶσιν
ἔσω ἐς τὴν μήνιγγα, ἥ τε ἄνω μοῖρα τοῦ ὀστέου καὶ ἡ κάτω, ἰητρεύοντι
ὡσαύτως τὸ ἕλκος ὑγιὲς τάχιστα ἔσται, καὶ τὰ ὀστέα τάχιστα ἐπάνεισι
τὰ ἐσφλασθέντα ἔσω.

18. Τῶν δὲ παιδίων τὰ ὀστέα καὶ λεπτότερά ἐστι καὶ μαλθακώτερα διὰ τοῦτο, ὅτι ἐναιμότερά ἐστι καὶ κοῖλα καὶ σηραγγώδεα καὶ οὔτε πυκνὰ οὔτε στερεά. καὶ ὑπὸ τῶν βελέων ἴσων τε ἐόντων καὶ ἀσθενεστέρων καὶ τρωθέντων ὁμοίως τε καὶ ἧσσον τὸ τοῦ νεωτέρου παιδίου καὶ μᾶλλον καὶ θᾶσσον ὑποπυΐσκεται ἢ τὸ τοῦ πρεσβυτέρου καὶ ἐν ἐλάσσονι χρόνῳ· καὶ ὅσα ἂν ἄλλως μέλλῃ ἀποθανεῖσθαι ἐκ τοῦ τρώματος, ὁ νεώτερος τοῦ πρεσβυτέρου θᾶσσον ἀπόλλυται.

2 Ἀλλὰ χρή, ἢν ψιλωθῇ τῆς σαρκὸς τὸ ὀστέον, προσέχοντα τὸν νόον
πειρᾶσθαι διαγινώσκειν, ὅ τι μὴ ἔστι τοῖσιν ὀφθαλμοῖσιν ἰδεῖν καὶ γνῶ-
25 ναι, εἰ ἔρρωγε τὸ / ὀστέον καὶ πέφλασται ἢ εἰ μοῦνον πέφλασται καὶ εἰ
3 ἕδρης γενομένης τοῦ βέλεος πρόσεστι φλάσις ἢ ῥωγμὴ ἢ ἄμφω ταῦτα. καὶ
ἤν τι τούτων πεπόνθῃ τὸ ὀστέον, ἀφεῖναι τοῦ αἵματος τρυπῶντα τὸ
ὀστέον σμικρῷ τρυπάνῳ φυλασσόμενον ἐπ' ὀλίγον· λεπτότερον γὰρ τὸ
ὀστέον καὶ ἐπιπολαιότερον τῶν νέων ἢ τῶν πρεσβυτέρων.

252 19. Ὅστις δὲ μέλλει ἐκ τρωμάτων ἐν κεφαλῇ ἀποθνήσκειν | καὶ μὴ δυ-
νατὸν αὐτὸν ὑγιᾶ γενέσθαι μηδὲ σωθῆναι, ἐκ τῶνδε τῶν σημείων χρὴ τὴν
διάγνωσιν ποιεῖσθαι τοῦ μέλλοντος ἀποθνήσκειν καὶ προλέγειν τὸ μέλλον
2 ἔσεσθαι. πάσχει γὰρ τάδε· ὁπόταν τις ὀστέον κατεηγὸς ἢ ἐρρωγὸς ἢ πε-

4–5 γίνεται] *cf.* Hipp. De locis in hom. 32: VI 324,6sq. L. 10 ὑποφύεται – διπλόης] *cf.* Cels. Med. VIII 3,10; 4,21: CML I, p. 377,1; 382,6sq. Orib. Coll. med. rel. XLVI 9,4: CMG VI 2,1, p. 219,7sq.

1 ἀφίεται V: ἀφίεται *in* ἀφίσταται *corr.* N 2 αὐτέου V: *corr. Erm.* δ' *add. Kollesch et Nickel* ἐν *add. Kollesch et Nickel* 2sq. τῷ – ἀφίσταται *del. Scal.* 8 κινδεύειν V: *corr.* Ho 9 εἰκὸς – χαλάσαντος *del. Erm.*: εἶδος πρῶτον χαλάσαντα *Corn.*: κως πρώτου χαλάσαντος *Scal.*: οἴδεος πρῶτον χαλάσαντος *Littré*: *cruces posui* 13 διαπύθη V: *corr.* Ho2 14 ποιήσειεν] πυήσηται V: ποιήσηται Ho2: ποιήσει *Erm.*: *corr. Kühlewein* 19 σηραιτώδεα V: οὐ σκληρώδεα Ho2: οὔτε σκληρώδεα *Ald.*: οὔτε σηραγγώδεα *Frob.*: *corr. Littré* 27 εἰ^{II} *post* καὶ^{I} *colloc.* V, *trsp. Erm.* 30 ἐπ' ὀλίγον] τὴν μήνιγγα *Reinh.*

come like a potsherd, separates most readily from the rest of the bone, which
contains blood and is living. But bone that, on its own, has become bloodless
and dry in the midst of living bone with good blood supply (also) separates
readily.

17. Cases in which the bones are crushed in, out of their normal posi-
tion, and are comminuted or severed with very wide separation are less dan-
gerous, as long as the membrane is intact. And, in cases of depressed, com-
minuted fracture, the greater the number of fractures and the wider their
separation, the less dangerous they are and the more easily they lend them-
selves to removal. It is not necessary to trephine any such cases or to risk try-
ing to extract the fragments of bone before they rise up on their own ... They 2
come up when flesh grows below them, and it grows up from the diploe of
the bone and from the healthy (bone) if the upper table alone of the bone is
necrotic. And in this way the flesh will grow from below and burgeon and
the bone fragments rise most rapidly if the wound is brought as rapidly as
possible to suppuration and made clean. And if the entire thickness of the 3
skull, with both its tables, outer and inner, is crushed in, onto the membrane,
it is by this same treatment that the wound will heal quickest and the bone
fragments that are crushed in will rise most rapidly.

18. The bones of young children are thinner and softer for this reason,
that they contain more blood and are hollow and porous and neither dense
nor hard. And in cases where the patients are wounded by weapons capable
of equal or less damage and (are wounded) to the same extent or less, the
(bone) of the younger child suppurates to a greater extent and more rapidly
than that of the older and for a shorter time; and of those who are destined,
in any case, to die of the wound, the younger perishes sooner than the older.

But, if the bone is laid bare of flesh, you must apply your mind to try to 2
discern what is impossible for the eyes to see and to determine whether the
bone has been fractured and crushed or only crushed, and whether, if a weap-
on *hedrē* is present, there is also crush-injury or fracture or both of these.
And if the bone has suffered any of these (injuries), let blood escape by per- 3
forating the bone with a small perforator, taking care (to check) at short in-
tervals, for the skull of young people is thinner and has less depth than that
of older persons.

19. When a patient is likely to die from his head wounds and cannot re-
cover his health or be saved, it is by means of the following signs that you
must make the diagnosis that he is going to die and predict what is going to
be. For (the patient) suffers the following: when, after recognizing that the 2

φλασμένον ἢ ὅτῳ γοῦν τρόπῳ κατεηγὸς ἐννοήσας ἁμάρτῃ καὶ μήτε ξύσῃ
μήτε πρίσῃ †μήτε δεόμενον, μήτε δὲ† ὡς ὑγιέος ἐόντος τοῦ ὀστέου, πρὸ
τῶν τεσσαρεσκαίδεκα ἡμερέων πυρετὸς ἐπιλήψεται ὡς ἐπὶ πολὺ ἐν χειμῶ-
νι, ἐν δὲ τῷ θέρει μετὰ τὰς ἑπτὰ ἡμέρας ὁ πυρετὸς ἐπιλαμβάνει. καὶ ἐπει-
δὰν τοῦτο γένηται, τὸ ἕλκος ἄχροον γίνεται καὶ ἐξ αὐτοῦ ἰχὼρ ῥεῖ σμι-
254 κρὸς καὶ τὸ φλεγμαῖνον ἐκτέθνηκεν ἐξ αὐτοῦ καὶ βλιχῶδες γίνεται | καὶ
φαίνεται ὥσπερ τάριχος χροιὴν πυρρόν, ὑπopέλιον. καὶ τὸ ὀστέον σφακε-
26 λίζειν τηνικαῦτα ἄρχεται καὶ γίνεται περκνόν, λεῖον ἐόν, / τελευταῖον δὲ
3 ἅπαν ὠχρὸν γενόμενον ἢ ἔκλευκον. ὅταν δ' ἤδη ὑπόπυον ᾖ, ἐπὶ τῇ γλώσσῃ
φλύκταιναι γίνονται καὶ παραφρονέων τελευτᾷ. καὶ σπασμὸς ἐπιλαμβάνει
τοὺς πλείστους τὰ ἐπὶ θάτερα τοῦ σώματος· ἢν μὲν ἐν τῷ ἐπ' ἀριστερὰ
τῆς κεφαλῆς ἔχῃ τὸ ἕλκος, τὰ ἐπὶ δεξιὰ τοῦ σώματος ὁ σπασμὸς λαμβάνει·
ἢν δ' ἐν τῷ ἐπὶ δεξιὰ τῆς κεφαλῆς ἔχῃ τὸ ἕλκος, τὰ ἐπ' ἀριστερὰ τοῦ σώμα-
τος ὁ σπασμὸς ἐπιλαμβάνει. εἰσὶ δ' οἳ καὶ ἀπόπληκτοι γίνονται, καὶ οὕ-
τως ἀπόλλυνται πρὸ ἑπτὰ ἡμερέων ἐν θέρει ἢ τεσσάρων καὶ δέκα ἐν χειμῶ-
νι. ὁμοίως δὲ τὰ σημεῖα ταῦτα σημαίνει καὶ ἐν πρεσβυτέρῳ ἐόντι τῷ τρω-
4 ματίῃ καὶ ἐν νεωτέρῳ. ἀλλὰ χρή, εἰ ἐννοοίης τὸν πυρετὸν ἐπιλαμβάνοντα
καὶ τῶν ἄλλων τι σημεῖον τούτῳ προσγενόμενον, μὴ διατρίβειν, ἀλλὰ πρί-
σαντα τὸ ὀστέον πρὸς τὴν μήνιγγα ἢ καταξύσαντα τῷ ξυστῆρι – καπυ-
ρὸν δὲ γίνεται καὶ εὔξυστον – ἔπειτα τὰ λοιπὰ οὕτως ἰητρεύειν, ὅπως ἂν
δοκῇ συμφέρειν πρὸς τὸ γινόμενον ὁρῶν.

20. Ὅταν δ' ἐπὶ τρώματι ἐν κεφαλῇ ἀνθρώπου ἢ πεπριωμένου ἢ
ἀπριώτου, ἐψιλωμένου δὲ τοῦ ὀστέου οἴδημα ἐπιγένηται ἐρυθρὸν καὶ ἐρυ-
256 σιπελατῶδες ἐν τῷ προσώπῳ καὶ ἐν τοῖσιν ὀφθαλμοῖσιν | ἀμφοτέροισιν ἢ
τῷ ἑτέρῳ – καὶ εἴ τις ἅπτοιτο τοῦ οἰδήματος, ὀδυνῷτο ⟨ἂν⟩ – καὶ πυρε-
27 τὸς ἐπιλαμβάνῃ καὶ ῥῖγος, τὸ δὲ ἕλκος αὐτὸ / ⟨τά⟩ τε ἀπὸ τῆς σαρκὸς κα-

5–7 ἰχὼρ ῥεῖ σμικρὸς ... καὶ φαίνεται ... ὑποπέλιον] *cf.* Hipp. Coac. praenot. 491: V 696,16sq. L. 6 βλιχῶδες] Erot. Voc. Hipp. collect. B 8: p. 28,10–14 Nachmanson schol. *in* Orib. Coll. med. rel. XLVI 23,3: CMG VI 2,1, p. 234,27 7 ὑποπέλιον] *cf.* Erot. Voc. Hipp. collect. Π 41: p. 72,7–10 Nachmanson Gal. Ling. s. dict. exolet. Hipp. explic. Π: XIX 129,7–9 K. 8 περκνόν] Erot. Voc. Hipp. collect. Π 43: p. 72,12 Nachmanson 9 ὑπό-πυον] *cf. supra,* p. 84,6 9sq. ἐπὶ – γίνονται] *cf.* Orib. Coll. med. rel. XLVI 23,3: CMG VI 2,1, p. 234,27 13sq.] *cf.* Hipp. Epid. V 28: V 228,2–4 L. 14 ἀπόπληκτοι γίνον-ται] *cf.* Hipp. Coac. praenot. 490: V 696,5sq. L. 18 διατρίβειν] Erot. Voc. Hipp. collect. Δ 12: p. 33,7 Nachmanson 23 ἐψιλωμένου – ἐρυσιπελατῶδες] *cf.* Hipp. Aphor. VII 19: IV 582,4 L. 25sq. καὶ[I] – ῥῖγος] *cf.* Hipp. Epid. V 16: V 216,2sq. L.

1 μὴ ἐννοήσας *Littré*: ἀγνοήσας *Reinh.* 2 *ante* μήτε[II] *add.* ὡς *Mart.* μήτε[II] – δὲ] ὡς μὴ δεόμενον, καὶ *Corn.*: ὡς μήτε δεόμενον μήτε δὲ *Mart.*: δεόμενον, μεθῇ δὲ *Littré*: *cruces posui* 5 γίνεται *e* γένηται *(?) corr.* V ῥέοι V: ῥέει N: *corr. Kühlewein* 6 βλιχῶδες *sec. Erot. scr. Erm.*: γλισχρῶδες V 8 λεῖον ἐόν] λευκὸν ὂν *coni. Maniaud,* λί-αν *Corn.* 9 ἀπάνωχρον V: *correxi; v. Index Hippocraticus, s. v.* ἔπωχρος, ὠχρός, ἅπας *(Addenda et corrigenda)*: „fort. leg. ἅπαν ὠχρόν": ἔπωχρον Ho[2] ᾖ] ἢ V: *corr. Corn., Foes. in adn.* 10 γίνωνται V: *corr.* C ἐπιλαμβάνη V: *corr.* Ho 13 τὰ] τὸ V: *corr. Ald.* 16 τρώματι ἢ V: *corr. Erm.* 17 εἰ *om.* V, *add.* Ho[2] ἐννοίης V: *corr.* N
19 καπυρὸν] εὔπριστον *Frob.* 25 ἂν *addidi* 26 ἐπιλαμβ[ά~] V: ἐπιλαμβάνη[οι] P: ἐπι-λαμβάνοι *Littré* τά *add. Reinh.* τε] τὸ *Foes.*

bone has been injured, either broken or crushed or at any rate in some man-
ner injured, (the doctor) errs and neither scrapes nor trephines ... as if the
bone were sound, fever will, as a rule, seize the patient within fourteen days
in winter, and in summer fever seizes him after seven days. And when this oc-
curs the wound becomes discolored and a small amount of serous discharge
flows from it and the inflamed tissue dies out of it and it becomes glutinous
and looks like salted fish, its color a livid red. Then the bone begins to ne-
crose, and, while remaining smooth, it becomes dark-colored and finally turns
entirely pale yellow or off-white. But when it has begun to suppurate, blisters 3
occur on the tongue and the patient dies delirious. And in most cases convul-
sion seizes the parts of the other side of the body: If the wound is on the left
side of the head, convulsion seizes the right side of the body, and if the
wound is on the right side of the head, convulsion seizes the left side of the
body. There are some patients who also become apoplectic, and in this condi-
tion they die within seven days in summer or fourteen in winter. These signs
have the same meaning, both in the older patient and in the younger. So if 4
you observe that fever is seizing (the patient) and that any of these other
signs accompanies it, do not waste time, but trephine the bone down to the
membrane or scrape down with the rasp – the bone becomes brittle and easy
to abrade – and then manage the rest of the medical treatment in a manner
that seems appropriate in view of the circumstances.

20. When, in the case of a head wound in which the patient has or has not been trephined but the bone is denuded, there occurs a red, erysipelas-like swelling of the face and one or both eyes – and the swelling may well be painful when touched –, and fever seizes (the patient), and chills, but the

λῶς ἔχῃ ἰδέσθαι καὶ τἀπὸ τοῦ ὀστέου καὶ τὰ περιέχοντα τὸ ἕλκος ἔχῃ κα-
λῶς, πλὴν τοῦ οἰδήματος τοῦ ἐν τῷ προσώπῳ, καὶ ἄλλην ἁμαρτάδα μηδε-
μίαν ἔχῃ τὸ οἴδημα τῆς ἄλλης διαίτης, τούτου χρὴ τὴν κάτω κοιλίην ὑπο-
2 καθῆραι φαρμάκῳ, ὅ τι χολὴν ἄγει. καὶ οὕτω καθαρθέντος ὅ τε πυρετὸς
ἀφίησι καὶ τὸ οἴδημα καθίσταται καὶ ὑγιὴς γίνεται. τὸ δὲ φάρμακον χρὴ
διδόναι πρὸς τὴν δύναμιν τοῦ ἀνθρώπου ὁρῶν, ὡς ἂν ἔχῃ ἰσχύος.

21. Περὶ δὲ πρίσιος, ὅταν καταλάβῃ ἀνάγκη πρῖσαι ἄνθρωπον, ὧδε
γινώσκειν· ἢν ἐξ ἀρχῆς λαβὼν τὸ ἴημα πρίῃς, οὐ χρὴ ἐκπρίειν τὸ ὀστέον
πρὸς τὴν μήνιγγα αὐτίκα. οὐ γὰρ συμφέρει τὴν μήνιγγα ψιλὴν εἶναι τοῦ
ὀστέου ἐπὶ πολὺν χρόνον κακοπαθέουσαν, ἀλλὰ τελευτῶσά πῃ καὶ διεμύ-
δησεν. ἔστι δὲ καὶ ἕτερος κίνδυνος, ἢν αὐτίκα ἀφαιρῇς πρὸς τὴν μήνιγγα
2 ἐκπρίσας τὸ ὀστέον, τρῶσαι ἐν τῷ ἔργῳ τῷ πρίονι τὴν μήνιγγα. ἀλλὰ χρὴ
258 πρίοντα, | ἐπειδὰν ὀλίγου πάνυ δέῃ διαπεπρίσθαι καὶ ἤδη κινῆται τὸ
ὀστέον, παύσασθαι πρίοντα καὶ ἐᾶν ἐπὶ τὸ αὐτόματον ἀποστῆναι τὸ
ὀστέον. ἐν γὰρ τῷ διαπριωτῷ ὀστέῳ καὶ ἐπιλελειμμένῳ τῆς πρίσιος οὐκ ἂν
28 ἐπιγένοιτο κακὸν οὐδέν· λεπτὸν γὰρ / τὸ λειπόμενον ἤδη γίνεται. τὰ δὲ
λοιπὰ ἰᾶσθαι χρή, ὡς ἂν δοκῇ συμφέρειν τῷ ἕλκει.

3 Πρίοντα δὲ χρὴ πυκινὰ ἐξαιρεῖν τὸν πρίονα τῆς θερμασίης εἵνεκα τοῦ
ὀστέου καὶ ὕδατι ψυχρῷ ἐναποβάπτειν. θερμαινόμενος γὰρ ὑπὸ τῆς περι-
όδου ὁ πρίων καὶ τὸ ὀστέον ἐκθερμαίνων καὶ ἀναξηραίνων κατακαίει καὶ
μέζον ποιεῖ ἀφίστασθαι τὸ ὀστέον τὸ περιέχον τὴν πρῖσιν ἢ ὅσον μέλλει
ἀφίστασθαι. καὶ ἢν αὐτίκα βούλῃ ἐκπρῖσαι [τὸ] πρὸς τὴν μήνιγγα, ἔπειτα
ἀφελεῖν τὸ ὀστέον, ὡσαύτως χρὴ πυκινά τε ἐξαιρεῖν τὸν πρίονα καὶ ἐν-
αποβάπτειν τῷ ὕδατι τῷ ψυχρῷ.

4 Ἢν δὲ μὴ ἐξ ἀρχῆς λαμβάνῃς τὸ ἴημα, ἀλλὰ παρ' ἄλλου παραδέχῃ
ὑστερίζων τῆς ἰήσιος, πρίονι χρὴ χαρακτῷ ἐκπρίειν μὲν αὐτίκα τὸ ὀστέον
πρὸς τὴν μήνιγγα, θαμινὰ δὲ ἐξαιρεῦντα τὸν πρίονα σκοπεῖσθαι καὶ ἄλ-
λως καὶ τῇ μήλῃ πέριξ κατὰ τὴν ὁδὸν τοῦ πρίονος. καὶ γὰρ πολὺ θᾶσσον
5 διαπρίεται τὸ ὀστέον, ἢν ὑπόπυόν τε ἐὸν ἤδη καὶ διάπυον πρίῃς. καὶ πολ-
λάκις τυγχάνει ἐπιπόλαιον ἐὸν τὸ ὀστέον, ἄλλως τε καὶ ἢν ταύτῃ τῆς κε-
φαλῆς ᾖ τὸ τρῶμα, ᾗ τυγχάνει λεπτότερον ἐὸν τὸ ὀστέον ἢ παχύτερον.
ἀλλὰ φυλάσσεσθαι χρή, ὡς μὴ λάθῃς προσβαλὼν τὸν πρίονα, ἀλλ' ὅπῃ
29 δοκεῖ πάχιστον εἶναι τὸ ὀστέον, ἐς τοῦτο αἰεὶ ἐνστηρίζειν τὸν / πρίονα,
260 θαμινὰ σκοπεόμενος καὶ πειρᾶσθαι ἀνακινέων τὸ ὀστέον | ἀναβάλλειν, ἀφ-

2sq. ἁμαρτάδα ... διαίτης] *cf.* Hipp. Epid. IV 20: V 158,20 L. 3sq. χρὴ – φαρμάκῳ] *cf.* Hipp. De ulc. 3: VI 404,11sq. L. 11 κίνδυνος – 12] *cf.* Cels. Med. VIII 3,7: CML I, p. 376,12sq. Orib. Coll. med. rel. XLVI 11,12: CMG VI 2,1, p. 220,26sq. 18sq.] *cf.* Cels. Med. VIII 3,7: CML I, p. 376,5–7 Orib. Coll. med. rel. XLVI 11,11: CMG VI 2,1, p. 220,23sq. 26 χαρακτῷ] Gal. Ling. s. dict. exolet. Hipp. explic. X: XIX 154,8 K. 29 ὑπόπυόν] *cf. supra,* p. 84,6

1 ἔχῃ[I]] ἔχοι V: *corr. Reinh.* ἰδέσθαι *del. Scal.* 3 ἔχοι V: *corr. Reinh.* 8 περιῆς V: *corr. Scal.* 13 ὀλίγου] υ *e* ν *correct. (?) in* V κινέεται V: κινέηται *Foes.*: *corr. Kühlewein* 15 διαπρίω τῷ V: *corr.* P 20 ὁ *om.* V, *add.* N 22 τὸ *deleverit Corn.*: *secl. Kollesch et Nickel* 32 τὸν] τὴν V: *corr. Ald.*

wound itself, as regards both flesh and bone, appears healthy and the tissues
around the wound are healthy, except for the swelling of the face, and the
swelling has not been complicated by any other error in the rest of (the pa-
tient's) regimen, in this case you should purge the bowel with a medicine to
draw off bile. After (the patient) has been purged in this way the fever re- 2
leases its hold and the swelling subsides and the patient gets well. But this
medicine must be given with an eye to the patient's vigor, to the strength he
has.

21. Concerning trephination, when necessity compels you to trephine a
patient, here is what you must know: if you trephine, having undertaken (the
patient's) care from the beginning, you should not excise the bone down to
the membrane straightaway. For it is not good for the membrane to be bare
of bone and subject to damaging exposure for a long time; otherwise it may
finally become macerated. And there is also another danger, that, if you tre-
phine down to the membrane and at once remove the bone, you may, in the
procedure, damage the membrane with the trephine. Rather, during trephina- 2
tion, when the bone lacks a very little of being sawn through and can already
be moved, you should stop trephining and let the bone separate on its own.
For in the case of bone which is sawn through but lacks some trephining no
harm will occur, since the bone left (undivided) is now thin. The rest of the
treatment should be that which seems appropriate to the wound.

When trephining it is necessary to remove the trephine frequently on ac- 3
count of the heat transmitted to the bone and to dip it in cold water. For the
trephine, heated by rotation, in turn, by heating and drying the bone, scorches
it and causes more of the bone surrounding the trephination site to separate
than would normally do so. If you want to trephine down to the membrane
immediately, and then remove the bone, you must, in the same way, take the
trephine out frequently and dip it in cold water.

If you do not take on (the patient's) care from the beginning, but receive 4
it from another (physician) and so are behind schedule in the medical treat-
ment, then, with a sharp-toothed trephine, you must immediately saw through
the bone down to the membrane, but frequently removing the trephine to in-
spect, with the probe as well as in other ways, around the path of the tre-
phine. For the bone is much more rapidly sawn through if you operate when
it has already begun to suppurate and is purulent through and through. And it 5
often happens that the skull has little depth, especially if the wound is in that
part of the head where the bone is more thin than thick. But you must guard
against careless application of the trephine, and always fix the trephine firm-
ly in the bone at the site where the bone seems thickest, inspecting it fre-
quently, and try, by rocking it back and forth, to lift the bone out; once the

ελὼν δὲ τὰ λοιπὰ ἰητρεύειν, ὡς ἂν δοκῇ συμφέρειν τῷ ἕλκει πρὸς τὸ γινόμε-
νον ὁρῶν.
6 Καὶ ἢν ἐξ ἀρχῆς λαβὼν τὸ ἴημα αὐτίκα βούλῃ ἐκπρίσας τὸ ὀστέον ἀφ-
ελεῖν ἀπὸ τῆς μήνιγγος, ὡσαύτως χρὴ πυκινά τε σκοπεῖσθαι τῇ μήλῃ τὴν
περίοδον τοῦ πρίονος καὶ ἐς τὸ παχύτατον αἰεὶ τοῦ ὀστέου τὸν πρίονα
7 ἐνστηρίζειν καὶ ἀνακινέων βούλεσθαι ἀφελεῖν τὸ ὀστέον. ἢν δὲ τρυπάνῳ
χρῇ, πρὸς δὴ τὴν μήνιγγα μὴ ἀφικνεῖσθαι, ἢν ἐξ ἀρχῆς λαμβάνων τὸ ἴημα
τρυπᾷς, ἀλλ' ἐπιλιπεῖν τοῦ ὀστέου λεπτόν, ὥσπερ καὶ ἐν τῇ πρίσει γέγρα-
πται [ἢν ἐξ ἀρχῆς λαμβάνων τὸ ἴημα πρίεις].

1 *post* ἕλκει *duo fragmenta libri Hipp. De aere aquis locis in* V *inserta sunt:* ὅτι – ἐγγένηται *(CMG I 1,2, p. 46,5–50,16) et* τοῦ – λιθιῶντες *(p. 28,3–46,5); cf. supra, p. 19* πρὸς – 8 γέγραπται *om.* N 2 ὀρρὸν V: *corr. A. Coray, Traité d'Hippocrate des Airs, des Eaux et des Lieux, Paris 1800, vol. II, p. 138sq.* 7 χρή V: *corr. Foes. in adn.* δὴ] δὲ V: *corr. Reinh.:* γε *Erm.* 9 ἢν – πρίεις *punctis del.* Ho[2]: *seclusi*

bone is removed, administer the rest of the medical treatment as seems appropriate to the wound in view of the circumstances.

If you take on the medical care (of the case) from the beginning and 6
want to trephine through the bone immediately and to remove it from the membrane, then in the same way you must frequently examine the circular course of the trephine with the probe and always fix the trephine in the thickest part of the bone and use back-and-forth movements in an attempt to
remove the bone. But if you use a perforator, do not penetrate through to the 7
membrane, in case you take on the medical care from the beginning and you do use a perforator, but leave intact a thin layer of bone, as has been written in regard to trephining.

COMMENTARY

P. 62,3: The Latin translation of De capitis vulneribus by Fabius Calvus (see above, p. 44) begins with the following sentences which have no equivalent in the Greek manuscript tradition: Capitis quidem vulnera nulla contemnito: nam saepe cutis sola contusa, scissa, recisave ferro, vel alia re, nisi diligenter, quadamque reverentia tractetur, cureturque, sanguinis coactione non expurgata, vel alia quavis re neglecta, vulnere recrudescente molestiam non parvam, et quandoque febrem adducit, magnumque negocium medico facessit: languenti vero mortis periculum portat, sed multo magis calvaria perfracta, proscissa, praecisave, cerebrique tuniculae: quae singula nisi medicus caute, perite, diligenterque tractet, et curet, languentibus mortem saepius accelerat, de quibus omnibus et alibi diximus, et hic cumulatius retractamus. Primo quidem capite modo aliquo percusso, quid percusserit petito, et si detur, perspicito, quid cum percussus fuit, laesus fecerit, percunctator et rimator.

Cornarius in his Latin translation of the treatise (see above, pp. 45–46) begins with a passage that provides the same material with different wording: Nullum capitis vulnus leviter contemni debet. Saepe enim cutis sola contusa ferro, aut alia aliqua re, si non diligenter, aut cum quadam cautione curetur: veluti si sanguis concretus non expurgetur: aut aliud quiddam negligatur: ulcus incrudescens non parum molestiae exhibet, et aliquando etiam febrem inducit: et medico quidem negotia, aegroto vero periculum non minus affert. Verum hoc multo magis contingit, si calvaria, et cerebri membranae rumpuntur. Quare si non singula haec diligenter medicus curaverit, saepe mortis causa existit. Et de his quidem omnibus etiam alibi diximus, sed et nunc dicendum est. Primum igitur capite vulnerato interrogare oportet: per quid vulneratum sit. Deinde quid homo fecerit, quum vulneratus fuit. Postea qua parte vulnus inflictum sit.

In the preface to his Latin edition Cornarius points out that an introductory section of De capitis vulneribus, which is present in the (Latin) editions, is lacking in the Greek printings. The only relevant Latin editions are those of 1525 and 1526 with the translation of Calvus. This is confirmed by a handwritten note of Cornarius in his copy of the Aldine Hippocrates (see above, p. 46 n. 1), fol. 191^{v} on the outer margin under the title of the treatise. This note refers to a passage in Greek and in his hand preceding the printed text: Calvus Interpres horum verborum sententiam hoc loco expressit, quem integrum habuisse videtur, quum in veteribus exemplaribus quae vidimus in totum defuerit. usque ad verba τῶν ἀνθρώπων αἱ κεφαλαὶ. From this it appears that Cornarius too was aware of no equivalent of this passage in the Greek manuscripts, but that he nonetheless accepted the fact that Calvus had translated an authentic text and this led him to change the material available only through Calvus into a more elegant literary form in his own translation.

The final step in Cornarius' philological efforts was his attempt to reconstruct from the revised Latin version the supposed original Greek text. He then entered this Greek passage in his copy of the Aldine. For this he used the space of 18 lines, between the treatise title and the beginning of the text, left free by the publishers of the Aldine, apparently in recognition of the fact that Calvus' translation pointed to additional text in that place. This Greek passage obtained by reverse translation is the following: τῶν τῆς κεφαλῆς τρωμάτων οὐδὲν εὐκαταφρόνητόν ἐστι· πολλάκις γὰρ τὸ δέρμα μόνον θλάσθεν (sic) ἢ διὰ σιδήρου ἤ τινος ἄλλου, εἰ μὴ ἐμμελῶς τε καὶ μετά τινος εὐλαβείας θεραπεύοιτο, οἷον αἵματος συμπεπηγότος μὴ καθαιρομένου, ἤ τινος ἄλλου ἀμελουμέμου, τὸ ἕλκος ὠμότερον γενόμενον οὐ σμικρὰ ἐνοχλεῖ, καί ποτε καὶ πυρετὸν ἐπιφέρει, καὶ ἰητρῷ μὲν πράγματα παρέχει, τῷ κάμνοντι δὲ κίνδυνον οὐχ ἧττον. ἀλλά γε τοῦτο πολὺ μᾶλλον γίνεται, ἐὰν τὸ κρανίον τε καὶ αἱ μήνιγγες ῥήγνυνται, ὥστε εἰ μὴ ἕκαστον τούτων ἐμμελῶς ὁ ἰητρὸς ἰήσεται, πολλάκις θανάτου αἴτιον γίνεσθαι· καὶ περὶ μὲν τούτων πάντων ἀλλαχοῦ εἰρήκαμεν, ἀλλὰ καὶ νῦν λεκτέον. πρῶτον μεν οὖν κεφαλῆς τρωθείσης ἀνέρεσθαι δεῖ δι' οὗ τρωθῇ, εἶτα τὶ ποιῶν ὤνθρωπος, τετρωμένος εἴη (in marg.: ἔπειτα ἐπὶ τινὸς μέρεος τὸ τρῶμα ῇ. [ἐπὶ – ῇ deleted] vel ὅπη τῆς κεφαλῆς ἔχῃ τὸ τρῶμα) καὶ γὰρ

This passage was printed in slightly altered form and with philologically inadequate revision by Petrequin, pp. 434–436.

The vocabulary in this passage confirms that it was not part of the original treatise and was, in fact, a later composition. In it the word κρανίον occurs, referring to the vault of the skull, whereas in the treatise itself κρανίον is found only once (p. 64,25) and in that instance it refers to the entire skull in a description of the tempero-mandibular joint. In the numerous references to the vault of the skull in De capitis vulneribus the author uses either κεφαλή or ὀστέον. Also, the word δέρμα and the plural αἱ μήνιγγες occur nowhere in De capitis vulneribus. σάρξ is used invariably for "scalp" and the singular μῆνιγξ for "dura mater". The plural "meninges" reflects a later stage of anatomical knowledge and nomenclature, where the dura mater and the pia mater together are referred to as "the meninges" (see below, pp. 97–98, the note to p. 62,24).

P. 62,3 οὐδὲ – 21: The word ῥαφή is among the earliest examples of technical, medical vocabulary. A word that, in common parlance, meant "seam" or "stitching" was appropriated by physicians and anatomists for the irregular, stitch-like seams or junctions of the cranial bones, a very fitting comparison. By the 5th c. the medical use of the term had been widely accepted and was in use not only by medical writers but by philosophers and natural historians, e.g. Plat., Tim. 76 a; Arist., Hist. anim. III 7: 516 a 18–20. Even historians and playwrights used the word freely, e.g. Herod. IX 83,2 and Eur., Phoen. 1159–1160; Suppl. 503. The word is so appropriate and became so well established that it has persisted, through Latin, as the word for "cranial suture" in the modern Western tongues.

The description of the cranial sutures in De capitis vulneribus, however, does not reflect normal cranial anatomy. The author describes the sutures as seen on the superior surface of the skull by an observer directly above it. He describes four arrangements:

1. If the skull has a prominence in front, the sutures appear as the letter T, the shorter suture transverse (= coronal suture), posterior to the prominence, and the longer suture in the midline (= sagittal suture), extending to the neck;

2. If the skull has a prominence posteriorly, the arrangement is the reverse, the shorter suture situated transversely anterior to the prominence (= lambdoid suture) and the longer suture extending in the midline to the forehead (= sagittal suture);

3. If there is a prominence both anteriorly and posteriorly, the sutures appear as the letter H, the shorter (= sagittal suture) in this case being in the midline and terminating at either end in a longer suture (= coronal and lambdoid sutures);

4. If there is a prominence at neither end, the sutures appear as the letter X, one extending to the temple on either side (= coronal suture), the other longitudinally in the midline (= sagittal and persistent metopic sutures).

Accurate description of the cranial sutures came late. Celsus, stating that neither the number nor the position of sutures is fixed, describes their usual arrangement, omitting the coronal suture (Med. VIII 1,2–3: CML I, p. 363,9–17). Rufus of Ephesus accurately describes the sutures "in most cases" and says that names had been recently applied by Egyptian doctors, poorly versed in Greek (De corp. hum. part. appellat. 130–133: pp. 150,9–151,4 Daremberg-Ruelle; De oss. 3: pp. 186,6–187,1 Daremberg-Ruelle). And even Galen, while giving their usual arrangement in heads with prominences both front and back, then describes the variations, comparing them to letters, as the author of De capitis vulneribus (De oss. ad tir. 1: II 740,1–741,9 K.).

The description of sutures in De capitis vulneribus is not only inaccurate but also too neat, too formulaic (e.g. absence of anterior prominence means absence of anterior suture). It sounds like an attempt at "rational" explanation of anatomical variation and smacks of philosophy, not anatomy. By contrast, the rest of De capitis vulneribus, including the description of the diploe and of the relative hardness and softness of the various parts of the skull, is basically accurate and empirical; a practical, practising surgeon is sharing his knowledge on diagnosis and treatment of skull injuries with other physicians. Writing at a time when the surface anatomy of the skull had not been well studied, he may have decided to preface his discussion with his "school notes" on sutures. Whatever its source, this description of cranial sutures does not reflect the reliance on observation and experience seen in the rest of the treatise.

P. 62,10: αἰεί appears several times, in similar context, in this section on anatomy (pp. 62,13; 64,1). Its intent is probably to indicate that the description given is of normal anatomy, the arrangement a surgeon should expect to encounter.

P. 62,12 πρὸ – ἐπικαρσίη: ἐπικάρσιος can take the genitive, and so, without πρὸ (πρὸ om. B) the sentence could be translated, "the shorter line is situated transverse to the prominence". However, the coronal suture is normally transverse to the longitudinal axis of the skull. The sense of this sentence must be to indicate where the suture is situated in relation to the prominence, not how. Therefore, πρὸ is necessary.

P. 62,23. 24: To the extent that the prefix ὁμο- in the word ὁμόχροια retains its own meaning, it indicates the smoothness and evenness of the skin (see Herod. I 74,6), the smooth surface of the cornea (see Hipp., De carn. 17,4: p. 18,10 Deichgräber = VIII 606,16 L.) or the sameness of color (see Arist., Meteora I 5: 342 b 20). In the present case it describes the evenness of the outer and inner tables of the skull, which, because of their compactness, differ from the porous bone between them. This description is of a cross section of the skull, with progression from the densest layers, outer and inner, where the bone appears uniformly compact, to the diploe, a region of vascular spaces divided by thin bony trabeculae, lying between the two dense layers. These layers, the outer and inner tables, are readily discernible, but they measure only a millimeter or so in depth. Their appearance, therefore, on cross section is not nearly so impressive as the smooth, hard outer and inner surfaces of the skull. This factor, added to the descriptions of Herodotus and of De carnibus, led to the acceptance here of the translation "even surface". Except for the solitary example in De carnibus the word ὁμόχροια is found nowhere else in extant Greek medical literature. Also the use later in De capitis vulneribus of another word, μοῖραι, for "tables" (p. 86,14) suggests that ὁμόχροια in De capitis vulneribus is a descriptive term rather than an attempt to expand and refine technical medical vocabulary. In later medical writings the inner and outer tables are referred to with the expressions λεία καὶ πυκνὴ ὀστοῦ λεπίς (Gal., De usu part. IX 1: II 5,20–21 Helmr. = III 690, 9–10 K.), ἐπιφάνεια τῶν ὀστῶν (Gal., Meth. med. VI 6: X 445,6 K.) and πυκνὴ ἐπιφάνεια (sc. ὀστέου) (Heliod. ap. Orib., Coll. med. rel. XLVI 9,2. 4: CMG VI 2,1, p. 219,2–3. 6–7; Paul. Aeg. VI 90,2: CMG IX 2, p. 137,8).

P. 62,24 μήνιγγι: In De capitis vulneribus the word μῆνιγξ is always singular and, with one exception (p. 80,18), always occurs in passages where the meaning "dura mater" satisfies the context. The plural does not appear; no reference is made to the pia mater; and no word other than μῆνιγξ is used of the dura.

The surgeon Heliodorus uses μῆνιγξ for the dura with the same assurance as the author of De capitis vulneribus (see e.g. Orib., Coll. med. rel. XLVI 11,1. 12. 23: CMG VI 2,1, pp. 219,26. 28; 220,27; 221,23). Galen confirms that, by his time, physicians were accustomed to calling the pia mater λεπτὴ μῆνιγξ and to reserving the term μήνιγγες for the exclusive use of the membranes around the brain (De anat. administr. IX 2: II 716,5–13 K.).

The dura mater is a tough, glistening, opaque, greyish, fibrous membrane, varying from approximately one millimeter to two millimeters in thickness. The pia is a delicate, filmy, transparent membrane, carrying the cerebral blood vessels, extending into all the sulci and fissures, and adherent to the brain. Two membranes could hardly appear more different than the dura and the pia. The dura is a substantial layer, distinct, separable from the skull for most of its extent, and tough, requiring a sharp object to penetrate it; the pia, by contrast, is filmy, insubstantial, difficult to separate from the brain and to isolate as a separate anatomical entity. The dura is a surgeon's membrane, the pia an anatomist's. The dura requires incision or suturing; the pia is insignificant surgically. Therefore, it is not surprising that a physician like the author of De capitis vulneribus, caring for patients with skull fractures and performing trephination, should be content with the term μῆνιγξ; the dura alone of the meninges requires surgical evaluation and treatment.

P. 62,25 ἀποχωρέον – 64,1 αἰεί: If the passage suggests increasing porosity as one passes from the outer surfaces toward the interior of the substance of the skull, then it must be noted that such a description is not accurate and does not concur with modern anatomical terms. The outer and inner tables vary from 1 mm or more in thickness, depending on the part of the skull and the individual, and are separated by the diploe which appears just as porous directly beneath the tables as at its center. The tables have fairly distinct inner surfaces and the diploe does not vary in porosity depending on its distance from either table.

P. 64,4 καὶ – 6 αὐτῶν: The manuscript reading ὅμοια was changed to ὁκοῖα, the emendation of Martin, by Littré, Ermerins and Reinhold. However, as Petrequin points out, the comparison to a sponge has just been made, and ὅμοια sustains this, describing fleshy areas which, as in sponges, contain liquid that can be expressed by pressure. This description of the diploe is essentially correct. It consists of vascular spaces which are irregular and variable in size and shape, separated by thin bony trabeculae, extending toward the interior of the bone from the outer and inner tables and intersecting one another at irregular angles. In most areas of the diploe these vascular spaces are lined by only a single layer of endothelium and so lack the usual vascular tubes that are seen in arteries and veins. The architecture of the diploe does resemble that of a sponge with its small, irregular cavities. Also the blood in the diploe gives it a "fleshy" appearance, quite unlike the dense, smooth, relatively avascular, grey-white surface of most bone. And the bony trabeculae separating the vascular spaces are so thin that they are easily broken by pressure from trephine or finger, thus opening vascular spaces and allowing blood to escape. Some of these vascular spaces are fairly round and so resemble the more typical blood vessels, φλέβια.

P. 64,9 συμπάσης – 10 βρέγμα: συμπάσης τῆς κεφαλῆς τὸ ὀστέον refers to the vault of the skull and does not include the facial bones, in particular the nasal bones, which are thinner than any part of the skull vault.

P. 64,13 τῶν τε τρωσίων – 14 ἧσσον: The use in this passage of the nominative case for the wounded, independent of the subject of the sentence, is not exceptional; corresponding construction occurs in other places in the treatise where similar thoughts are expressed: pp. 64,30–32; 78,6–7.

P. 64,17 ἐξίσων τε ἐόντων τῶν τρωμάτων ⟨...⟩: The fact that the phrase refers back to the situation described in lines 13–14 suggests that here too a double modifier had been supplied for the noun (τῶν τρωμάτων), just as, in both cases, in regard to the injuries, the alternative possibilities ὁμοίως τε ... καὶ ἧσσον are listed. In the transmitted wording the nonconnective τε (line 17) arouses suspicion that is removed if the loss of the second member introduced by καί is accepted. Littré added the words καὶ ἡσσόνων after τρωμάτων. The parallel passages in which at least two-membered expressions are used in the description of comparable situations (lines 13–14. 31; pp. 78,6–7; 86,20) makes it even more likely that, with regard to the injuries in this passage as well, the author used the formular καὶ ἐλασσόνων.

A further problem with the passage is ἐξίσων. The adjective ἔξισος is otherwise unknown. ἐξισόω is fairly common and ἔπισος, though rare, is documented. Ermerins has therefore, in reliance on the phrase ἀποθανεῖσθαι ἐκ τοῦ τρώματος (line 19), altered the text, ἐξ ἴσων τε ἐόντων τῶν τρωμάτων ... ἀποθνήσκει ὁ ἄνθρωπος. But with this change the καὶ before ὁμοίως becomes unintelligible, since in this case it no longer connects two parallel members. The fact that, in the form ἐξίσων, the word transmitted in the manuscripts constitutes a hapaxlegomenon – in the Index Hippocraticus the word ἔξισος is listed as dubia lectio – is no basis not to retain it in the text.

P. 64,26–27 φλὲψ ... κοίλη τε καὶ ἰσχυρή: The vessel referred to is the superficial temporal artery (cf. M.-P. Duminil, Le sang, les vaisseaux, le cœur dans la Collection hippocratique. Anatomie et physiologie, Paris, 1983, p. 30). Although arteries and veins appear to be differentiated in some Hippocratic works (e.g. De artic. 45: II 171,18–19 Kw. = IV 190,7 L.; De carn. 5,2: p. 6,27–28 Deichgräber = VIII 590,10–11 L.), the word φλέψ usually means "blood vessel", referring to either artery or vein. This nonrestrictive use of the term is characteristic of fifth-fourth century usage. For a concise account of early Greek concepts of the vascular system see H. v. Staden, Herophilus. The art of medicine in early Alexandria, Edition, translation and essays, Cambridge, 1989, pp. 169–181. κοίλη describes the liquid-carrying capacity of the vessel and ἰσχυρή probably the force of the blood in this small vessel.

P. 64,28 κορυφῆς: Used of the head, κορυφή means "top" or "vertex". Throughout the Hippocratic Corpus it has this general sense, e.g. ὑπὲρ τοῦ ὠτὸς ἄνω πρὸς κορυφὴν τὸ τρῶμα ἦν, Epid. VI 4,5: V 308,9–10 L., and συνάψαι τοὺς ἱμάντας κατὰ τὴν κορυφήν, De artic. 33: II 152,3 Kw. = IV 152,2 L. It is not a well-defined anatomical term. Head trauma in early Greek medical literature is described with reference to regions of the head rather than to cranial bones. The regions are μέτωπον, βρέγμα, ἰνίον, κορυφή and κρόταφοι. κορυφή is the medial and superior part of both βρέγμα and ἰνίον bilaterally.

P. 64,31 ἐόντων: The unanimously transmitted reading ἁπάντων makes no sense. On the basis of parallel passages (lines 13–14. 17; p. 86,20) Littré replaced it with ἐόντων which one would expect in this location.

P. 64,32: Littré properly deleted the word μειόνων (μιονος B) as nonsensical since context requires that the wounds or weapons be equal or larger, not smaller.

P. 66,4 ἐλάσσων ταύτῃ τῆς κεφαλῆς ὁ ἐγκέφαλος ὕπεστι: While the accuracy of this statement can be challenged, it appears to represent a view held even more strongly by Aristotle (Hist. anim. I 7: 491 a 34–b 1). The part of the head referred to by ταύτῃ corresponds roughly to the area posterior to the lambdoid suture. The skull here overlies the occipital lobes above the tentorium and the cerebellum below it. In both regions the healthy brain lies fairly close to the dura with little apparent subarachnoid space. However, on dissection of the posterior fossa, the area below the tentorium, the subarachnoid space is very evident in places, especially in the large cisterns around the midbrain, pons and medulla, and, in particular, in the cisterna magna on the inferior surface of the cerebellum. These large reservoirs of cerebrospinal fluid may account for this statement in De capitis vulneribus.

P. 66,6–7 ἐν χειμῶνι πλείονα χρόνον ζῇ ὤνθρωπος ἢ ἐν θέρει: This point is made twice in De capitis vulneribus (see also p. 88,15).

In this passage, dealing with infection, the obvious implication is that death occurs sooner in warm weather due to putrefaction. Galen, as transmitted by Oribasius (see above, p. 38), makes an observation which supports this assumption: προσήκει κατὰ τὴν πρώτην ἡμέραν ἐκκόπτειν τὸ πεπονθὸς ὀστοῦν, εἰ καὶ μὴ πᾶν, ἀλλὰ τό γε κατεπεῖγον, καὶ μάλιστα ἐν ὥρᾳ θερινῇ· κατὰ ταύτην γὰρ ἀναβάλλεσθαι τὴν χειρουργίαν οὐ χρή, διότι θᾶττον ἴσμεν ἐν ταῖς θερμαῖς ὥραις σηπόμενα πάντα (Coll. med. rel. XLVI 21,30: CMG VI 2,1, p. 231,1–5). The likeliest explanation of this statement is necrotic tissue. The low-velocity injuries of antiquity were especially apt to abrade, crush and avulse soft tissue (skin, pericranium, muscle). It must have been common for head wounds to contain not only dirt but also blood clots, detached fragments of other soft tissue or badly crushed soft tissue. Such tissue, deprived of a normal blood supply, would, of course, rot, and, like all dead flesh, rot faster in warm weather. This necrosis and suppuration would then serve as a nidus for spread of infection to bone and deeper tissues. In view of the practical, empirical nature of most of the advice in De capitis vulneribus, the warning that death occurs more quickly in summer than in winter most likely describes the response to contamination and necrosis in undebrided or inadequately debrided wounds.

P. 66,9–12: The construction Αἱ δὲ ἕδραι ... ἐκ τουτέων ὁ θάνατος οὐ γίνεται is an anacoluthon in the form of a nominative in suspense.

P. 66,9: Hedrē means "seat", and, as used here of skull injury, describes the mark made by a weapon as it strikes the skull, a groove or hole, sometimes with the weapon still "seated" in the skull. This type of injury is discussed in ch. 7, where it is defined, ἕδρη γὰρ καλεῖται, ὅταν μένον τὸ ὀστέον ἐν τῇ ἑωυτοῦ φύσει τὸ βέλος στηρίξαν ἐς τὸ ὀστέον δῆλον ποιήσῃ, ὅπου ἐστήριξεν (p. 70,4–5). In modern nosology such injuries are considered fractures, rather than the "bite" of a weapon, and the term would not, in any case, define a group of patients requiring treatment different from that of other skull fractures, except for extraction of the weapon if still in situ.

While a missile or the edge of a weapon can produce a skull defect in its own shape, such an injury can occur only when impact is at considerable velocity. Low velocity impact produces either no fracture or a nondescript linear or comminuted fracture of the sort seen with blunt injuries. No doubt spears and swords could, with the right angle and the right speed, cleave the skull and leave a defect suggesting their shape; certainly arrows and other missiles could. E. W. Marsden, Greek and Roman artillery. Historical development, Oxford, 1969, pp. 95–96 and plate 5, reports a skull, probably of the

1st c. A.D., with a square temporal defect that corresponds exactly to catapult bolts found near it.

Because there is no comparable modern term, the Greek word ἕδρη has simply been transliterated in this edition.

P. 66,10 ῥωγμῆς τε καὶ φλάσιος καὶ ἔσω ἐσφλάσιος: According to the author of De capitis vulneribus the conditions designated as ῥωγμή, φλάσις and ἔσφλασις, along with ἕδρη, constitute the major types of skull injury. They are grouped together, as seen in passages lines 19–20 and pp. 70,23–72,1, under the general terms κάτηγμα, κάτηξις, expressions which otherwise are used for bone fracture.

By ῥωγμή the author means a crack-like fracture in the skull vault. ἔσφλασις occurs when a fractured section of skull is displaced inward from its normal position (see p. 68,18–21). φλάσις, on the other hand, is a form of injury in which the skull is damaged, either superficially or deeply, but without necessarily sustaining a fracture (see p. 68,7–12). The author himself points out that this type of injury cannot, at least immediately after its occurrence, be diagnosed on examination (p. 68,14–16).

Differentiation of the various types of injury leads to difficulties in adequate translation of the expressions. The problem begins with the words κάτηγμα and κάτηξις. In their usual medical context these words are used of bony fractures with obvious loss of continuity. In De capitis vulneribus the author clearly states that φλάσις, one of the types of κάτηγμα / κάτηξις, does not constitute a fracture. Therefore he has redefined the words and they no longer mean, in this context, either "fracture" or "break". That the author does not bother to further define them suggests that he assumed his audience was already acquainted with this usage. In any case, in the context of De capitis vulneribus, κάτηγμα and κάτηξις are best translated by the general term "injury".

Apart from three examples, occurring in context similar to that of De capitis vulneribus (De locis in hom. 32: VI 324,8. 9 L.; cf. above, p. 55; Prorrh. II 14: IX 38,1 L.), in the Corpus Hippocraticum the expression ῥωγμή, referring to skull injuries, is found only in the present text. In one other place it is used with the common meaning "tear / rupture" in reference to the eye (Prorrh. II 19: IX 46,13 L.). In keeping with its general, nonmedical, usage in the treatise De capitis vulneribus the word ῥωγμή in reference to the skull means "crack" or, in medical terminology, "linear fracture" (the synonym ῥῆξις is also used, pp. 76,16. 18. 19. 23; 80,29; 82,3). It is not surprising that fractures of the smooth extensive convex surface of the skull elicited terms different from fractures of the relatively small irregular surfaces of the long bones. The surface of the skull resembles that of a vessel and a linear fracture in the skull vault resembles a crack in a ceramic pot (cf. Sor., De signis fract. 2,1: CMG IV, p. 155,6–8) or a fissure in the dry level earth or in a smooth piece of wood (cf. Arist., Hist. anim. V 28: 556 a 4–6; IX 9: 614 b 15), an appearance very different from that of an open long bone fracture. While physicians in antiquity would have seen skull fractures, only rarely would a physician see an exposed long bone fracture other than the sharp end of a grossly displaced humerus, femur or other long bone protruding through torn muscle and skin. The difference in appearance of the two types of fracture is so great that the existence of a special term for skull fracture became quite reasonable.

As used in De capitis vulneribus the word φλάσις (related to φλᾶν, "crush") must be regarded as a technical term, redefined to describe a blunt head injury in which there is no initial evidence of skull damage. This concept was difficult for physicians later on in antiquity who tended to regard φλάσις as a pediatric diagnosis, explained by the elasticity of the immature skull, allowing reversion to normal shape after injury (see e.g. Heliod. ap. Orib., Coll. med. rel. XLVI 17,1: CMG VI 2,1, p. 224,12–14; Gal., De morb. causis 11: VII 38,12–39,5 K.). Uncertainty regarding the term's meaning has persisted; the translation favored by modern editors, "contusion", "Quetschung", "contusione" (Littré, Petrequin, Adams, Withington, Fuchs, Vegetti), is inadequate because the current medical use of "contusion" is restricted to soft tissue and describes a response to trauma whose main feature is bruising, i.e. the force of trauma has been sufficient to burst small blood vessels, but not sufficient to break the overlying tissue (skin, muscle).

The term φλάσις had, however, a usefulness that far exceeded its awkwardness. The author of De capitis vulneribus treats head injuries almost exclusively as skull injuries. Apart from brief mention of impaired consciousness (pp. 76,8–9; 82,12–13) and contralateral seizures (p. 88,10–11) he acknowledges no neurologic abnormalities, not even such gross signs as weakness and paralysis. He realises, in a general way, the importance of the brain in maintaining vital functions (p. 64,9–23), but otherwise does not discuss the brain. No mention is made of such major pathology as cerebral laceration and contusion or intracerebral hemorrhage. The dura mater, too, figures only rarely in his advice (pp. 84,19–23; 86,6; 88,19; 90,8–12. 22. 27; 92,7), usually as a barrier to avoid. Subdural and epidural hematomas, both obvious and treatable conditions, are not recognized (except for a doubtful reference: p. 86,29). Such a system, ignoring the major life-threatening complications of head injury and attempting to regulate treatment and to determine prognosis on the basis of skull injury alone, has an obvious and serious defect; it has no reasonable way to account for the morbidity and mortality due to intracranial injury. There would have been many patients whose clinical course could not be explained by the degree of damage seen on inspection of the exposed skull. Those cases in which the patients did poorly but had no apparent skull damage must have been the most vexing. Of the five types of skull injury listed in De capitis vulneribus, only φλάσις and 'injury elsewhere than the scalp wound' (p. 70,18) were available for such cases. φλάσις, therefore, very likely became a catch-all diagnosis for patients who did poorly in the absence of demonstrable skull damage. In this edition φλάσις is translated "crush-injury", in an attempt to convey some sense of the Greek word and yet specify no particular pathology.

According to the definition given in ch. 6 (p. 68,18–21) ἔσφλασις is the inward displacement of damaged skull; it is not itself fractures, but it is accompanied by fractures and cannot occur without fracture. For modern physicians, the primary pathology is fracture, and the diagnosis is "depressed fracture". In this translation in order to maintain the linguistic connection between the expressions ἔσφλασις and φλάσις the equivalent term "depressed crush-injury" is used for ἔσφλασις.

P. 66,16 ἕλκος: The transmitted βέλος arouses suspicion. The phrase τὸ – γενόμενον indicates a special case of the general statement in lines 13–14, πανταχοῦ τῆς κεφαλῆς τοῦ ἕλκεος γενομένου; therefore, one expects the subject in this instance as well to be ἕλκος, as Ermerins conjectured. Also the possible confusion of the words ἕλκος and βέλος, which in this passage are repeatedly used in alternation, is obvious from a paleographic point of view.

P. 66,21 τῇ ῥωγμῇ ἐν: Both manuscripts transmit a corrupt text (τῆς ῥώγμης ἐν B: τῇ – ἐν om. V) which was corrected by Kühlewein; cf. p. 68,26: τῇ τε ῥωγμῇ καὶ φλάσιν προσγενέσθαι ἀναγκαῖόν ἐστιν. The omission in V probably represents an unsatisfactory attempt at correction, if one assumes that the common ancestor of B and V already contained the error seen in B.

P. 66,22 ἥνπερ ῥαγῇ: Because of the repetition several times in lines 21–22 that the bone is broken, Ermerins objected to the pleonasm and changed ἥνπερ to ᾗπερ ἄν. However, pleonasm is characteristic of the style of De capitis vulneribus, as seen again in a similar passage, p. 68,26–28, and so alteration of the text is not called for.

P. 68,6: The extensive supplements given in the apparatus represent the editors' intentions to create a stricter parallelism among the possible types of simple skull fractures and to produce agreement with the similar statements in lines 10–11. The additions, however, are not required by the sense of the passage and such strict parallelism is not an invariable aspect of the author's style.

P. 68,7: Here and, with the exception of p. 76,21, in all its other occurrences in De capitis vulneribus φύσις means "normal position". It is used with the same meaning in the orthopedic treatises of the Corpus Hippocraticum (e.g. De fract. 15; 40; 44: II 72,11; 104,2; 107,4 Kw. = III 474,2; 546,13; 554,20 L.).

P. 68,13 τὴν ἰδέην: While the plural, ἰδέαι, is consistently used in this treatise as designation of subordinate classifications under the major types (τρόποι) of skull injury (even in the preceding sentence, line 12), the word here in the singular is to be taken in its original sense as "shape". Grammatically, τὴν ἰδέην, as τὸ μέγεθος, is an accusative of respect, modifying the preceding relative pronoun.

P. 68,16: The phrase ἑκὰς ἐοῦσαί τε refers to cases in which the fracture occurs at a site other than the external wound; cf. p. 70,18. For ἑκάς see also above, p. 36 n. 1.

P. 68,25–28 ῥωγμήν: The sense of the passage is this: 1. a hedrē occurs, 2. a fracture may accompany a hedrē, 3. if a fracture occurs together with a hedrē, then necessarily a crush-injury also occurs where the hedrē and fracture are and also in the bone surrounding the hedrē and fracture.

P. 68,26–28 τῇ τε ῥωγμῇ ... καὶ ῥωγμὴ ... ἡ ῥωγμὴ ... τὴν ῥωγμήν: For the pleonastic, repetitive style cf. p. 66,21–25. The loss of τῇ τε ῥωγμῇ in B could have been caused by the preceding dative ἑδραιηι.

P. 70,1–6 τέταρτος οὗτος τρόπος ... πέμπτος οὗτος τρόπος ... ⟨ἕκτος οὗτος τρόπος.⟩: Under τρόποι the author of the treatise groups the major types of skull injuries (see p. 66,19) which by his reckoning amount to seven (p. 66,25 εἷς οὗτος τρόπος; line 19 ἕβδομος οὗτος τρόπος). In keeping with this plan ῥωγμή, φλάσις and ἔσφλασις are dealt with in chapters 4–6 as τρόποι 1–3 (pp. 66,25; 68,8. 22). But, deviating from this plan in this passage, the different forms of hedrē are presented as τρόποι, although one would expect hedrai as a group to represent a single τρόπος. And the presentation in this case proceeds, contrary to expectations[1], from the most complicated through the less complicated to the simplest types of injury: hedrē in combination with ῥωγμή and φλάσις is numbered type 4, and hedrē in combination with φλάσις alone type 5, while hedrē without any complication (lines 3–5) is not numbered. Since all the other τρόποι appear under numbers, the failure to give a number in this case (ἕκτος οὗτος τρόπος) must be imputed to the manuscript tradition. Paleographically the loss of text is easiest to explain before ἐν δὲ τῷ τρόπῳ, line 6. And this is also the site where the number of the item just described would be placed, since in the following passage the various forms (ἰδέαι) of types 4–6 are presented, an arrangement which corresponds to that elsewhere in the section where the presentation of the ἰδέαι follows the enumeration formula (... οὗτος τρόπος). On this basis the addition recommended by Ermerins seems justified.

P. 70,11 στόμα: As opposed to σχῆμα, the variant transmitted in V, the reading of B takes precedence as lectio difficilior. And στόμα with the meaning "point" or "edge" of a weapon, is supported elsewhere; see LSJ, s. v. III. 1.

P. 70,18 Ὀστέον – 19 τρόπος: The author of De capitis vulneribus gives the seventh type of skull injury no special name; he says only that this injury is elsewhere than the scalp wound. The same phenomenon is described by Celsus (Med. VIII 4,6: CML I, p. 378,20–25) and by Galen in an excerpt of his commentary on De capitis vulneribus preserved by Oribasius (Coll. med. rel. XLVI 21,8–9: CMG VI 2,1, p. 228,21–26); Galen says that this kind of fracture is called ἀποκόπημα by some more recent physicians.

A special term, ἀπήχημα ("echo"), existed, although perhaps not so early as De capitis vulneribus, for skull injury directly opposite the external wound (see Sor., De signis fract. 8: CMG IV, p. 156,11–13); it referred therefore to only one of the injuries possible in the category described in this passage. The strict definition of ἀπήχημα was challenged even in antiquity (see Paul. Aeg. VI 90,2: CMG IX 2, p. 137,10–19). Still, some modern commentators, e.g. Vidius and Petrequin, apparently influenced by ἀπήχημα, have, in discussing this passage, used the terms "contrafissura" and "contrecoup".

We now know: 1. that skull fracture may occur at sites other than that of impact, 2. that the force that produces it is the force of impact transmitted through the bone itself, not through brain and other soft tissue to the opposite side of the calvarium, 3. that most often such fractures occur in areas adjacent to the site of impact, and 4. that skull fracture may occur not only at a

[1] Because of this Reinhold and Kühlewein have transposed the passage p. 70,3 καὶ – 5 ἐστήριξεν (description of the simple hedrē) to the beginning of ch. 7, thereby destroying the arrangement of the author.

site other than that of the scalp wound, but without any scalp laceration at all. The term "contre-coup" is now used in cases of closed head injury where the clinical picture indicates brain dysfunction on the side opposite impact and the mechanism is thought to be the differential in acceleration-deceleration between brain and skull.

P. 70,21: ἐξελέγχειν has been taken here by some editors to refer to history-taking, the questioning of the patient by the physician, e.g. Foës ("ex eius percunctatione deprehendas"). However, the broader meaning, "investigate, examine, prove" has been given by others, e.g. Littré ("il n'est possible de reconnaître par aucune recherche") and Petrequin („il n'y a aucun procédé, à quelque recherche qu'on se livre, pour reconnaître"). This latter sense suits the context of the treatise better since the head-injured patient, sometimes dazed or comatose, cannot always respond to questioning. Indeed, the author of De capitis vulneribus uses ἐξελέγχειν later (p. 72,24) in this broader sense.

P. 70,23 κατήξιος: See above, p. 101, the note to p. 66,10.

P. 70,24 ἡ ῥωγμὴ ἡ ἀφανὴς ἰδεῖν: What sort of fracture is impossible to see? Skull fractures elsewhere than the scalp wound have just been excluded from medical help because the physician cannot determine the site of fracture. Presumably the author is referring here to the occasional fracture that is so fine that it is overlooked or to the fracture occurring in a suture. But another factor may account for this description: physicians knew fractures primarily as those with gross displacement, often with protrusion of jagged, bloody edges. By contrast, any linear skull fracture could be called "difficult to see". The distinctive term ῥωγμή, in itself, alerts the physician to expect something out of the ordinary; ἀφανής, applied to it, is a warning that the physician must be very careful to look for a subtler, less obvious, type of fracture.

P. 72,5 διακοπὴ γὰρ καὶ ἕδρη τωὐτόν ἐστιν: The same idea has already been expressed, if in somewhat different words, at p. 70,14–17 and the same words are used twice later, at pp. 76,3–4; 78,3–4. This formula and its two repetitions were deleted by Ermerins as supposed marginal glosses. But the entire treatise contains numerous repetitions, phrases and sentences, often repeated word for word. This appears to be a characteristic of its author. Moreover, the text used by Erotian contained this phrase at p. 76,4 where it is followed by φλᾷ δὲ οὐ μάλα (see above, p. 36).

P. 72,9 καὶ^II – 10 ἔχειν: The arrangements in B and V are: καὶ ην τουτο ην φαναι κινδυνευειν ... σαρκὸς ἔχειν B: κινδυνεύειν ... σαρκὸς καὶ ἣν τοῦτο ἧ φάναι ἔχειν V. Although the construction in the reading of V is grammatically possible, difficulties arise in regard to style and content: 1. The sentence begins abruptly without an introductory conjunction, 2. κινδυνεύειν must syntactically be dependent on χρὴ (line 6) and therefore is grammatically equivalent to the infinitives σκοπεῖσθαι (line 6) and καταμανθάνειν (line 8), which represent instructions to the doctor, while κινδυνεύειν, as an impersonal expression, states an objective circumstance, and 3. the doctor would be advised to diagnose skull injury before he could be certain. In contrast, the text in the arrangement of B, apart from the necessary supplement of a καὶ before ἔχειν, is correct in language as well as in content: the doctor is advised to inspect the wound, and, if the hair has been driven into it, then to state that there is a danger that the skull has been exposed and injured. With this construction both ψιλὸν εἶναι and ἔχειν τι σίνος rely on κινδυνεύειν. B's arrangement of the text is supported by parallel wording, pp. 78,27; 80,15–17.

P. 72,10 ψιλὸν ... τῆς σαρκὸς: Throughout De capitis vulneribus the concept of bareness, either of the skull or of the dura, is critical to diagnosis, as in this passage (cf. lines 13. 14. 20; pp. 76,10; 86,25), and to treatment (cf. pp. 78,27; 84,5. 26; 88,23; 90,9).

P. 72,13 καὶ ἢν – 14 εἰ δὲ μή: This use of a positive protasis without an apodosis, followed by an negative protasis, εἰ δὲ μή, is encountered elsewhere in the Corpus Hippocraticum, e.g. De diaeta acut. (spur.) 37 (14): I 166,14–15. 19–20 Kw. = II 472,5–474,1. 5 L.; De morbis II 15. 25: VII 28,17–18; 40,5 L.; De mul. nat. 8: VII 322,22–324,1 L.

The protasis καὶ ἢν – ⟨ἐόν⟩ makes an important distinction: bone may be bare, i.e. the soft tissue may have been stripped from it as a result of trauma, but in these cases the bone is not always and, in fact, often is not visible to the eyes. This occurs when the avulsed scalp falls back over the exposed skull or when blood clot or hair covers it. The author therefore states not only the primary condition, that the bone be laid bare, but also the secondary condition, that it remain visible on inspection.

P. 72,14: In addition to the probe mentioned in this passage (μήλη; cf. also the derivative μήλωσις) three other surgical instruments, used in the treatment of head injuries, are mentioned in De capitis vulneribus: the rasp (ξυστήρ; cf. also ξύειν, ἐπιξύειν, καταξύειν, ξύσις, εὔξυστος), the perforator (τρύπανον; cf. also τρυπᾶν) and the trephine (πρίων; cf. also πρίειν, διαπρίειν, ἐκπρίειν, πρῖσις, ἄπριστος, ἀπρίωτος, διαπριωτός). The use of a fifth instrument, the scalpel or knife, is indicated by the words τάμνειν, ἐπανατάμνειν and τομή. This stock of instruments may seem scanty, considering the nature of the surgical procedures described. But the author of De capitis vulneribus clearly did not intend to describe in a systematic way the surgical armamentarium, and when instruments are mentioned, it is incidental to the context. One can therefore assume that still other instruments could be used, without being mentioned in the text. For photographs and discussion of the instruments referred to see E. Künzl, Medizinische Instrumente aus Sepulkralfunden der römischen Kaiserzeit, Köln and Bonn, 1983 (Kunst und Altertum am Rhein 115), pp. 15–17; 20–21; 27–28.

P. 72,18 ἢν – 20 ὀστέου: In this part of the sentence the wording transmitted after ποιεῖσθαι in B and V, ψιλοῦ τε ἐόντος τοῦ ὀστέου, does not suit the required meaning, because the genitive absolute is coupled by τε with the clause introduced by ἢν, resulting in contradictory statements referring to the same bone. After the expression πολλῷ ἔτι μᾶλλον one expects a term of comparison and this is provided by the genitive absolute with Ermerins' addition of ἢ before ψιλοῦ and his correction of τε to γε.

P. 74,2 μᾶλλον – 3 ὅταν^II: In sections 1–3 of this chapter, the author classifies head injuries by mechanism: those inflicted by another person, by the patient's falling, and by something falling on the patient's head. The intent is to assist the doctor in assessing the likelihood of one or more of the types of skull damage discussed. Accordingly, in the first category, wounds due to another person, the doctor is told to pay attention to four factors: assailant's intent, angle of blow, assailant's control of his weapon and assailant's strength relative to the patient's.

The passage cited here presents several problems. The major manuscript readings are: ὁκοταν ἑτερος ὑφ' ἑτερου τιτρωσκόμενος επιτηδες τρωσαν βουλομενος· ἢ οκοταν ακεων καὶ οκοταν B: ὅταν ἕτερος ὑφ' ἑτέρου τιτρωσκόμενος ἐπίτηδες τρῶσαι βουλόμενος ἢ ὅταν V.

Both manuscripts show errors. τρωσαν B has arisen from the infinitive τρῶσαι (dependent on βουλόμενος) through a scribal error; ακεων B, as Littré has correctly seen, is another mistake in copying, here of the letters of ἀέκων (as the antithesis of ἐπίτηδες ... βουλόμενος). In V the passage after ὅταν^{I}, corresponding to the reading ακεων καὶ οκοταν B, has been omitted through homoioteleuton. But the wording that results after the elimination of these special errors still raises several problems: 1. ἕτερος lacks a finite verb; 2. τιτρωσκόμενος, βουλόμενος and ἀέκων can hardly refer to the same person; 3. ἢ ὅταν with the meaning demanded by context, "than when", implies a comparative antecedent.

As concerns a predicate for ἕτερος, a finite verb can be obtained by changing the participle τιτρωσκόμενος to τιτρώσκηται. For solution of the remaining problems[1] it must be made clear that in this passage an intentional wound appears to be contrasted to an unintentional wound, just as in the following statement (lines 3 καὶ ὅταν – 4 χωρίου) a blow from above is contrasted to a level blow. In view of this situation βουλόμενος and ἀέκων must refer to the attacker (ὑφ' ἑτέρου) and not to the injured (ἕτερος), with the grammatic consequence that the transmitted nominatives be changed to genitives. Therefore, in agreement with βουλομένου, the correction made by Scaliger, ἀέκοντος must replace ἀέκων. The parallelism of the statements suggests that ἢ ὅταν, corresponding to the formula μᾶλλον ἢ ὅταν (line 4), also was dependent on a μᾶλλον. Accordingly, to reconstruct the necessary sense, the superlative μάλιστα (line 2) must be corrected to μᾶλλον.

P. 74,6 πρός – 7 ὀστέον^{II}: The phrase is probably intended to alert the physician that, even if the only injury immediately apparent is to the soft tissue overlying the skull, still he should be alert, if the patient has fallen from a height onto a hard, blunt surface, to the possibility of serious head injury.

P. 76,3 ἐμποιεῖ – διακόψαν: The participle διακόψαν indicates that as subject to ἐμποιεῖ the singular τὸ βέλος is intended. Accordingly a double change in number is present here (line 1 plural τὰ βέλεα – line 3 singular – line 4 plural τὰ βέλεα). αὐτὸ refers to the preceding τὸ ὀστέον and is the accusative object of διακόψαν.

P. 76,3 διακοπὴ – 4 ἐστι: See above, p. 105, the note to p. 72,5.

P. 76,8 καὶ^{I} – 9 πέσῃ: The wording καὶ ἢν δῖνος, as transmitted in B, is

1 The textual emendations proposed for this passage by Littré and Petrequin are, in general, unsatisfactory because, in the one case, they consist of major alterations to the transmitted wording, and, in the other, they are connected with significant problems in interpretation.

preferable to the reading of V, καὶ δῖνος, because it results in the sensible pairing of stupefaction with darkening of vision and of vertigo with falling.

This is one of the few passages in De capitis vulneribus where neurologic signs and symptoms are mentioned. The treatise deals almost exclusively with skull injuries, rarely relating them to brain dysfunction. Here, however, is unequivocal evidence not only that alteration of consciousness was recognized as a possible consequence of head injury, but also that it was regarded as an index of severity (cf. p. 82,12–13).

With the same meaning as in this passage and at p. 82,12 σκότος otherwise is found within the Corpus Hippocraticum only in Epid. V 23: V 222,17 L. The verb σκοτοῦν is used in the same context in Epid. V 50; VII 32: V 236, 13; 402,1 L. σκότος and σκοτοῦν, used of vision, describe darkening of vision as an early and prominent feature of the whole physiologic event which results in loss of consciousness.

The author of De capitis vulneribus distinguishes clearly between σκότος and δῖνος. Other Hippocratic writers, however, use the compounds, σκοτόδινος (Aphor. IV 17: IV 506,11 L.; Prorrh. II 30: IX 62,21 L.; Epid. VII 84: V 442,2 L.) and σκοτοδινίη (Coac. praenot. 157: V 618,5 L.; De affect. 2: VI 210,9 L.; De prisca med. 10: CMG I 1, p. 43,3; De morbis II 4; 15; 18: VII 12, 12. 13; 28,4; 32,3 L.) which LSJ translates, "dizziness, vertigo", but which probably, in most instances, are intended to express darkening of vision as well as vertigo. From the modern point of view, the problem here is not only semantic but also conceptual. Vertigo and loss of vision are discrete symptoms, each with its own causes. However, in the common condition of syncope or fainting, loss of consciousness associated with sudden fall in blood pressure, there is an association of darkening of vision and loss of vision with a sensation of motion of surrounding objects. While this sensation is not true vertigo, it is similar and could be called δῖνος. The confusion persists in the present use of "dizzy" to describe everything from unsteadiness to a feeling of lightheadedness to actual vertigo. The Hippocratic writers, despite their limited knowledge of physiology, seem to have been more precise in their use of these words. σκότος and σκοτοῦν were used of darkening and loss of vision, δῖνος of vertigo, and the compounds, σκοτόδινος and σκοτοδινίη, of the confusing mixture of these symptoms seen commonly in syncope.

Galen's definition of σκοτόδινος confirms the force of both parts of the compound, σκοτόδινος δ' ἐστίν, ἐπειδὰν ἅμα περιδινεῖσθαι δοκῇ τὰ βλεπόμενα, ἥ τε διὰ τῆς ὄψεως αἴσθησις ἐξαίφνης ἀπολεῖται, δοκούντων αὐτῶν σκότος περικεχύσθαι (In Hipp. Aphor. comm. IV 17: XVII B 677,4–6 K.). However, in some later use the compounds and even σκότωμα and σκότωσις assumed the meaning of δῖνος and were used loosely for "dizziness", cf. e.g. Erot., Voc. Hipp. collect. Δ 11: p. 33,4 Nachmanson: δῖνος· σκότωσις, ὡς φέρεσθαι δοκεῖν τὰ ὁρώμενα. For fuller discussion of this see M. L. Hanson, Eye terms in Greek tragedy, Diss. Chapel Hill, 1987, pp. 301–310.

P. 76,11 χαλεπὸν – 14 ῥαφῇσιν: Concerning this passage, Littré properly points out that a hedrē which is obvious elsewhere in the skull may be difficult to see in the area of a suture and that, since a hedrē in the area of a suture may be difficult to recognize, the surgeon, examining a head wound in which a line that resembles a suture is exposed, must be aware of three possibilities: 1. the line is a hedrē, 2. the line is a suture, or 3. the line is both, i.e. a hedrē directly in the suture itself.

P. 76,14 συγκλέπτει: As its object γνώμην or ὄψιν must be understood; cf. the almost identical phrase, συγκλέπτουσι γὰρ τὴν γνώμην καὶ τὴν ὄψιν ... αἱ ῥαφαὶ (p. 78,1–2).

P. 76,17 ὡς – γινομένῃ: The readings of the major manuscripts are: ὡς ἐπι τόπου αυτησιν ἐν τησι ῥαφησι γινομενησι B: ὡς ἐπὶ τὸ πουλὺ αὕτη ἐν τῇσι ῥαφῇσι γινομένησι V. Both versions contain several errors. τόπου αυτησιν B has resulted from confusion of majuscules (ΛΥ 〉 ΑΥ) and incorrect separation of the words τὸ πουλὺ τῇσιν. The same source of corruption is responsible also for the reading αὕτη V; here, since it was not recognized that the paired letters αυ arose from λυ, the incorrect separation of words has been corrected only partially and που has been expanded to πουλὺ (cf. the same phrase ὡς ἐπὶ τὸ πουλύ V, line 19). The dative plural in B is explained just as the form γινομένησι, transmitted in B and V, as an error by attraction, caused here by τῇσι ῥαφῇσι. Since the participial form must agree with the article τῇ which is derived from the reading αὕτη in V, the dative plural must be changed to the dative singular. The reading τῇ ... γι(γ)νομένῃ was restored by Littré, although with different reasoning.

P. 76,25 οὔτε – 27 διαχαλάσῃ: Both major manuscripts provide an incorrect text: ουτε η απο εδρης του βελεος γενομενης ἐν τη ραφη· επειδαν ῥαγη καὶ διαχαλασηι· οὔτε ἢν φλασθεντος του ὀστεου κατα τας σαρκας ῥαγη καὶ διαχαλασθη B: ἦ, οὔτε ὑπὸ ἕδρης τοῦ βέλεος γενομένης ἐν τῇ ῥαφῇ· ἐπειδ' ἂν ῥαγῇ καὶ διαχαλάσῃ V.

The readings σαρκας and διαχαλασθη in B are obviously corrupt. σάρκας is not a sensible reading. If the fracture were beneath, i.e. covered by, soft tissue it would indeed be difficult to diagnose. The discussion here is of wounds in which the skull is exposed, ψιλωθὲν τὸ ὀστέον (line 10). διαχαλασθῇ seems unlikely in view of the διαχαλάσῃ of both B and V in the preceding phrase and of the intransitive use of διαχαλᾶν in the other places it occurs in De capitis vulneribus. In both instances the corrections of Littré have been accepted (ῥαφὰς and διαχαλάσῃ). The serious error in V consists of the omission, due to homoioteleuton, of the passage lines 26 οὔτε – 27 διαχαλάσῃ. The η (= ἤ) transmitted in B after οὔτε (line 25) might have been a later addition, referring to ῥῆξις (line 23) and probably inserted because, on account of the unusual location of the conjunction ἐπειδὰν (ἀπὸ – ῥαφῇ is part of the temporal clause), the true construction was not recognized. In V this addition was integrated into the text before οὔτε and as a subjunctive form connected with the preceding εὐμαρής.

P. 78,5 ἐς τὸ ὀστέον: Littré's restoration here is based on the parallel phrases, p. 74,6–7. 12. The phrase, πρὸς τὸ ὀστέον, in itself, is incomplete, requiring ἐς τὸ ὀστέον or αὐτὸ τὸ ὀστέον to express completion of the injury.

P. 78,14 οὐδὲ – ἥκιστα: This somewhat enigmatic phrase may well have been altered in transmission. De ulceribus, a treatise that shares much advice and many expressions with De capitis vulneribus (see above, pp. 53–54), permits the use of wine ("Ελκεα ξύμπαντα οὐ χρὴ τέγγειν, πλὴν οἴνῳ, De ulc.

1: VI 400, 2 L.), while proscribing the use of other topical medicines in wounds (Ἔλαιον δὲ καὶ ὅσα μαλθακώδεα ἢ ἐλαιώδεά ἐστι φάρμακα, οὐ ξυμφέρει τοῖσι τοιούτοισιν ἕλκεσιν, De ulc. 2: VI 404,4–5 L.).

P. 78,19 ἐκ – 20 ἐπιρροήν: There are two assumptions implicit in this passage. The first is that blood flowing into wounded tissue leads to swelling. The second is that the scalp does not have blood flow so great as that of the forehead and periorbital regions.

Neither of these assumptions is correct. First, when a wound is closed, i.e. when the skin in the area of trauma is intact, then rupture of blood vessels leads to swelling. However, when the skin is broken, blood escapes and edema is due largely to cell membrane damage with loss of intracellular liquid to the intercellular space. The vascular contribution to swelling is more often due to venous obstruction and diapedesis than to active bleeding into an open wound. Second, the blood supply to the scalp is rich. Scalp lacerations, including those of the vertex, bleed as vigorously as those of the forehead and periorbital areas. Nonetheless, the advice contained in this passage is sound and is based, as usual in this treatise, on accurate clinical observations. Wounds of the forehead and face do swell more than scalp wounds. The difference, however, is not in the blood supply but in the structure of the skin. The scalp is relatively thick, tight and dense, with less subcutaneous fat, while the skin of the face is thinner, softer, with more abundant and looser subcutaneous tissue. Facial skin, therefore, is readily distensible and more easily allows accumulation of extracellular, extravascular liquid. In view of these structural differences, poultices, to draw out edema fluid, and bandaging, to compress the looser tissue and so discourage swelling, are more beneficial to facial wounds than to scalp wounds. The author of De capitis vulneribus was aware that the scalp and facial skin respond differently to trauma. But he assumed, incorrectly, that the difference was due to blood supply. In short, the distinction made in this passage between scalp wounds and wounds in the forehead is valid, and the treatment prescribed is sensible.

P. 80,1 καὶ δ' αὖτε: This combination is a problem in several respects. Neither the direct pairing καὶ δέ nor the form αὖτε occurs elsewhere in prose. Numerous examples of the pairing δ' αὖτε occur in the Homeric epics, so possibly here there is an echo of epic language. The proposal that δ' αὖτε be taken as δαὖτε, crasis for δὴ αὖτε (so Denniston, p. 199; Index Hippocraticus, s. v. αὖτε), represents no convincing solution, since that form too is attested only in poetry and, moreover, is even rarer.

P. 80,3 τὰ – 8 ἕλκος: Incision and opening up are recommended for those head wounds in which the skull is exposed but the scalp laceration is not large enough to permit adequate examination of the skull. Two classes of wounds are considered, according to their shapes. The crucial characteristic, both in classifying the wound and in determining treatment, is described by the word ὑπόκοιλα. LSJ's definition, "slightly concave", for which this passage is given as the first example, is erroneous and misleading. While it is possible that the term could be applied to the external appearance of an area of crushed scalp, the meaning here is different and is clear from context. The physician is advised to incise and open up the cavity, τὸ κοῖλον. ὑπόκοιλα, therefore, means "hollow below" and is used to describe scalp which has been detached from the skull, creating a potential cavity between scalp and skull. Withington has properly used "undermined", the term generally applied to skin detached from deeper tissue. That the extent of undermining is great is specified by ἐπὶ πολύ. Although minor detachment of skin from underlying tissue is possible without a break in the skin, extensive detachment, of the sort described in this passage, implies an open wound. In both types of wound described here two conditions pertain: 1. the scalp is torn or lacerated, exposing the skull, and 2. the scalp is extensively undermined.

The distinguishing feature of the two types is their shape, one is linear and undermined to one side, ἐς πλάγιον, the other rounded and undermined on all sides. The treatment for both types is ἐπανατάμνειν, to incise and open up. The force of ἐπανα- is probably "elevate". The advice in De capitis vulneribus then is to incise the scalp over the undermined area, thus creating flaps which can be elevated so as to open up the wound, exposing its furthest limits. The treatment recommended for a wound undermined to one side is incision into the cavity; the treatment recommended for a rounded wound with undermining around its circumference is incision across the circumference.

The phrase ὥσπερ πέφυκεν ὤνθρωπος means "vertically", in a cephalocaudal direction (i.e. parallel to the long axis of the body), as opposed to "transversely" (cf. lines 28–29: κατὰ μῆκος τοῦ ἀνθρώπου, ὡς πέφυκε, καὶ αὖτις ἐπικάρσιον). A vertical extension of the wound achieves exposure of the base of the wound and also tends to avoid transection of the larger blood vessels.

In fact, blunt wounds are rarely symmetrically round. They are more often irregularly oval, with undermining which is also not concentric, but more in one direction than in others. When incision is necessary for proper debridement, it is usually made over the area where the undermining is most marked and, if possible, as an extension of the long axis of the wound. The rationale for treatment by incision as given in De capitis vulneribus is the basis for wound management even in this age of antibiotics; the entire wound, to its furthest corners, must be inspected and physically cleaned.

P. 80,11 σπασμὸς – 14 ἐπιλαμβάνει: In the early Greek medical literature σπασμός is a general term encompassing various phenomena; the word means an involuntary movement, varying from a cramp or mild spasm, to a twitch or jerk, to the sustained spasm of tetanus, to the clonic-tonic movements of a full-blown major motor seizure.

In De capitis vulneribus itself the lack of precise definition is seen. In the present passage σπασμός occurs as a result of surgical incision in the temple. The reference must be to a very specific injury in which there is an unstable comminuted fracture, probably with dural laceration, so that the pressure from incision of the skin and temporal muscle causes stimulation of the underlying motor cortex and a jerk of the contralateral extremities. It is possible that such stimulation of an already irritated cortex could precipitate a clonic-tonic seizure, but more likely the result would be a solitary jerk, or, with repeated bouts of pressure, repeated jerks. In ch. 19 (p. 88,4–14), however, where discussion is of infected head wounds with the occurrence of σπασμός on the side opposite the wound, the term (p. 88,10. 12. 14) certainly refers to major motor seizures.

The statement relating temporal incision to contralateral seizure is too general. As pointed out, that would be apt to occur only in cases where the fracture was unstable, with bone fragments easily displaced, and the dura lacerated as well. In most cases of temporal fracture the bone is fixed and the pressure of incision is not transmitted to the brain. However, the temporal bone is thin and can be shattered more easily than most of the other cranial bones. When this occurs and when the dura is lacerated at the same time, the temporal cortex is vulnerable. Although this is not a common situation, it could result in stimulation or damage to the motor cortex at surgery, either by the surgeon's pressing bone fragments into the brain or even lacerating it with the scalpel. This, in turn, could cause a spasm or jerk of the contralateral extremities, a dramatic consequence of surgical incision and one apt to be reported and attributed to injury in the area, rather than to the particular predisposing features of the wound.

P. 80,17 τομήν: The word τομή, transmitted in B (τομης), is appropriate here; it occurs earlier (pp. 78,24; 80,3) in this discussion. But the case required is accusative as present in V (τολίην). τομήν is credible as a cognate accusative, with τὸ μέγεθος an accusative of respect.

P. 80,18 ᾗ – 19 πέφυκεν: This clause probably describes the anatomy of the scalp as observed surgically. The scalp separates fairly readily from the skull in the plane of the areolar tissue just above the pericranium, a thin, tough fibrous membrane which is closely adherent to the skull and remains attached to the skull unless a special effort is made to incise it and scrape it free or unless it is torn loose, as in some fractures. μῆνιγξ, therefore, in this passage must mean "pericranium", which is not referred to elsewhere in De capitis vulneribus. The author's use here of the same word for pericranium as elsewhere for dura mater (see pp. 62,24; 84,19. 20; 86,6. 15; 88,19; 90,9 bis. 11. 12. 22. 27; 92,4. 7) is an example of the loose, nonspecific nature of early technical terminology.

P. 80,22 μάζῃ – ἀλφίτων: The fineness of the meal is an essential factor in producing a sticky, coherent poultice.

P. 82,3 μὴ – 4 ἐόντα: In this construction προσγένηται and λανθάνῃ depend equally on μὴ, although, as regards content, only λανθάνῃ can refer to μὴ, while πολλάκις ... προσγένηται must have expressed a causal or attributive relationship to ῥῆξις καὶ φλάσις: "lest ῥῆξις and φλάσις, because they (*or* which) frequently accompany hedrē". Despite the logical inconsistency in the train of thought the text should be retained in its transmitted form, because ἔπειτα, which follows, refers back to the preceding clause and so coordinates the verbs dependent on μὴ. Reinhold did not take this circumstance into account when he prepared the following emendation: μὴ, ἃ πολλάκις τῇ ἕδρῃ προσγεγένηται, ῥῆξις καὶ φλάσις ...

P. 82,6 καὶ ... μὴ: The ου δη, transmitted after καὶ in B, probably is best taken as οὐ δεῖ (as in N), and very likely represents a marginal gloss, intended to replace μὴ, and inserted in the wrong place. If this assumption is correct, the intervention in the text is based on a failure to recognize the construction in which a transition occurs from the impersonal expression to the imperative infinitive.

P. 82,14 δεῖ – 18 ἐπιξῦσαι: This passage contains a peculiarity of grammar. It begins with δεῖ and an accusative-infinitive construction, δεῖ ... δεύσαντα ... στεῖλαι, while the following infinitives ἐπιδῆσαι and ἐπιξῦσαι are combined exclusively with nominative participles. This situation has caused some editors to alter the text in an effort to achieve uniformity of construction. Littré, for instance, changes all the nominative participles to accusatives.

It is, however, quite likely that the author of De capitis vulneribus had in mind the type of construction seen often in recipes for medicines, where the verbs are frequently limited to nominative participles and infinitives, i.e. the main verb is an infinitive used as an imperative and the participles modify the understood nominative subject of the infinitive. He introduced this section on treatment with δεῖ and therefore placed the participle occurring before the infinitive in the accusative case. But then he reverted to the usual nominative participles and infinitive imperatives.

The advice given in this passage is sensible, and, as usual in De capitis vulneribus, reflects years, probably generations, of experience. Fine particles in solution will enter a fresh fracture, even one too thin to be readily seen otherwise. A linen dressing protects the wound from the coarse and irritating components of the poultice and bandage. Oil, applied over the linen, saturates it and so prevents its adhering to the wound surface and causing bleeding when removed. And the final bandage or dressing holds the poultice in place.

P. 82,23 φλάσις – 24 ξυστῆρος: φλάσις is further defined here as a cause of fracture of the outer table alone, a fracture so fine that it is detected only by uptake of the black contrast material. This is a rare condition but one in keeping with the general definition of φλάσις as physical damage invisible on routine examination.

P. 84,1 ἀλλὰ χρὴ: For the progressive use of ἀλλά in the Corpus Hippocraticum see Denniston, p. 21.

P. 84,8 περισφίγγηται: LSJ, giving this passage as example, translates περισφίγγω, pass., "contract, shrink", presumably in the sense of "pulled back around the periphery". This meaning accurately describes the behavior of inflamed scalp wounds where the deeper and looser layers of the scalp become more edematous than the tighter superficial layers, causing separation of the skin edges, often with exposure of the bone. This aspect of scalp inflammation is significant in the treatment of the wound and may be the aspect described by περισφίγγηται.

P. 84,8–9 πυρετῶδες ... πλέον: The gender of the adjectives could indicate that ὀστέον is the subject in mind. However, even though repetition of ideas is common in De capitis vulneribus, in this instance, where the same statement occurs in the following sentence, with ὀστέον as its subject, πυρετῶδες and πλέον are best taken as predicate neuters referring to injured soft tissue in general.

P. 84,12–15 κακὸν δὲ καὶ ὑγρήν τε εἶναι τὴν σάρκα ... χρὴ διάπυον μὲν ποιῆσαι τὸ ἕλκος ὡς τάχιστα. οὕτως γὰρ ... τάχιστ' ἂν καθαρὸν εἴη:

The same idea in very similar words is seen in ch. 17,2 (p. 86,13–14). Some degree of inflammation seems to have been considered inevitable, and the goal of medical therapy was to make that phase of wound reaction as brief as possible. In the theory of De capitis vulneribus, and very prominently in that of the Hippocratic treatise De ulceribus, wet wounds are considered diseased and dry wounds healthy. Galen reports that the medical regimen for cases of head injury assured good wound healing by making the wound dry and clean, ὡς ξηρὸν μὲν ἅπαν εἶναι τὸ χωρίον, ἕκαστον δὲ μέρος τῶν πεπονθότων ὀστῶν ἀκριβῶς καθαρόν (Gal., Meth. med. VI 6: X 446,9–11 K.); this regimen included ξηρὰ φάρμακα (ib., p. 445,15–16 K.).

P. 84,18 ὑπερσαρκήσειε: All wounds, surgical or traumatic, heal by the production of granulation tissue. In the space between skin edges blood and serum form a coagulum in which fibroblasts proliferate and capillary buds are formed. This friable, red fibrous tissue with its new blood vessels is granulation tissue. Under ideal circumstances its surface is covered by epithelial cells which migrate from the skin edges and restore skin continuity. Sometimes, however, especially in infected wounds and in wounds where skin edges are widely separated, granulation tissue grows exuberantly, above skin level. Such exuberant tissue, so-called "proud flesh", can interfere with epithelialization and thus with normal healing of the wound. That it was a common problem in the infected gaping wounds of antiquity is indicated by its mention by Celsus (Med. VIII 4,21–22: CML I, p. 382,8–9) and Archigenes (ap. Orib., Coll. med. rel. XLVI 25: CMG VI 2,1, p. 235,12–35).

P. 84,22 ξαίνηται: The readings of both B, ξαινηται, and V, ἐξαίρηται, are possible. ξαίνεσθαι may be used of bodies to mean "to be mangled, lacerated", and ἐξαίρεσθαι can mean "to swell". ξαίνηται, a word rarely found in medical context, has been retained as lectio difficilior.

P. 84,24–86,3: In this chapter the author points out that injured bone separates from normal bone once it has become bloodless and dry and that the process of drying occurs with the help of medications and with time. As in other sections (pp. 86,12–17; 88,17–21) the need for prompt treatment is emphasized. Here the surgeon is advised to treat the wound by cleansing and with medication in order to obtain the most rapid separation of the damaged bone (line 28 – p. 86,1), although it is pointed out that with time these changes may occur on their own (p. 86,2–3).

The text of the last two sentences in the section is corrupt. The manuscript reading τούτω instead of τοῦτο (line 30) arose from the associated corruption, ἀπεστρακὸς, ἐν, for ἀποστρακωθὲν (line 30), taking the dative; Ermerins' restoration of τοῦτο is accepted. ἀφίεται (p. 86,1), as middle voice with the meaning "free / loosen itself from" is uncommon, and therefore the more usual ἀφίσταται, the corrected reading of N, is accepted. The final sentence, as transmitted, lacks an adversative conjunction to set it off and contains a dative of uncertain function; both problems are paleographically easy to understand, the loss of a δ' and the omission of ἐν after a word ending in -ον. They have been restored: αὐτὸ ⟨δ'⟩ ἔξαιμον ... ξηρὸν ⟨ἐν⟩ τῷ ἐναίμῳ. αὐτὸ is construed as emphatic, with the meaning "by itself / on its own", i.e. without the use of medication.

P. 84,26 γενόμενον: Separation of exposed bone would not occur while the bone was in the process of becoming bloodless, as the manuscripts' γινόμενον would suggest, but rather after the bone had become bloodless. Therefore the correction of Ermerins has been accepted.

P. 86,6 ἐπὴν – ᾖ: This clause does remove from the group discussed those cases with dural laceration and therefore many that would also have damage to the brain. But significant pathology (subdural hematoma, brain hemorrhage and/or swelling) can occur with the dura intact and, in these cases, it is often evident through the dura. The force of ὑγιὴς here might be to exclude such serious trauma from the group of cases that are "less dangerous". However, such an important distinction would certainly call for more discussion, at the very least a description of the normal dura. Considering that no attention is given here or elsewhere in the treatise to distortion of the dura from underlying pressure or to its discoloration from subdural blood, it is likely that in this instance ὑγιὴς signifies nothing more than the integrity of the surface of the membrane.

P. 86,7 ἀκινδυνότερα – ἀφαίρεσιν: The same point is made in De locis in hom. 32: VI 324,6–8 L.: Κεφαλῆς κατήγματα· ἢν μὲν τὸ ὀστέον καταγῇ καὶ ξυντριβῇ, ἀκίνδυνον ... ἢν δὲ ῥαγῇ καὶ ῥωγμὴ ἐγγένηται, ἐπικίνδυνον. Extensively comminuted skull fractures, especially those with separation, and therefore mobility, of fragments, are easier to open up surgically. Also, because of the mobility of the fragments, readier drainage of blood is allowed from within the skull toward the surface and, compared to the intact skull with only a single linear fracture, a degree of decompression is provided. To this extent this section of De capitis vulneribus is accurate. It does not, however, address the most important aspect of head injury, that is, the severity of brain damage. Patients with extensively comminuted skull fractures often have injury to the underlying brain, even with the dura intact. It would be extremely bad judgement to consider such a patient at less risk than one with a simple, linear fracture and no evidence of brain damage.

P. 86,9: The phrase εἰκὸς πρῶτον χαλάσαντος is corrupt. Syntactically neither εἰκὸς nor the genitive participle suit the construction. χαλάσαντος lacks a noun or pronoun for which the intransitive meaning of the verb "become loose, subside" would be suitable, unless one accepts Littré's substitution of οἴδεος for εἰκὸς ("when swelling has first subsided") or supplies an understood ὀστέου, less likely because of the disagreement in number ("it is likely once it has become loose"). It is quite unlikely that these words represent the remnant of a more extensive original passage, since the following ἐπανέρχεται refers directly to the preceding ἐπανίῃ. Also the train of thought is complete in itself without the addition. Similar considerations may have caused Ermerins and following him Kühlewein as well (and perhaps also Littré, vol. X, pp. XXI–XXII) to delete the passage as a gloss.

P. 86,14–15 ἄμφω αἱ μοῖραι ... ἥ τε ἄνω μοῖρα τοῦ ὀστέου καὶ ἡ κάτω: μοῖραι refers to the dense, compact bone forming the outer and inner layers of the skull and enclosing the looser, more vascular diploe; cf. the anatomical description at pp. 62,22–64,2.

P. 86,29 αἵματος: Opening of the vascular spaces of the diploe does, as noted by the author (p. 64,5–6) result in some minor loss of blood, but not enough to be considered a therapeutic bloodletting. Since epidural hematomas are relatively uncommon, the reference here may be to the clinically insignificant amount of extravasated blood commonly associated with skull fractures.

P. 86,30 τρυπάνῳ: The perforator or auger has at its tip only one sharp point as opposed to the multiple cutting points of the trephine, and the bony opening produced, because of its conical shape, allows ready assessment of the depth of penetration. Also the surgeon does not have to maintain as precise an alignment of the instrument during penetration. For these reasons it was considered safer and easier to use than the trephine for pediatric cases in which the skull is thinner and the patient often less cooperative.

P. 86,35–88,1 κατεηγὸς ... κατεηγὸς: See above, p. 101, the note to p. 66,10.

P. 88,1 ἐννοήσας: Littré, considering the omission of surgical treatment the result of a mistake in diagnosis, has, in accord with the argument of Vidius (Chirurgia, p. 105), added the negative μὴ before ἐννοήσας. In the present case, however, the error referred to may well be one of treatment, not diagnosis: the physician recognizes the presence of an injury but does not operate. In this instance he is guilty of ignoring the guidelines of treatment put forward in the treatise, not of carelessness in diagnosis. The transmitted text should therefore be retained.

P. 88,2: The passage μήτε δεόμενον, μήτε δὲ represents a textual corruption whose emendation, as the proposals of earlier editors show, appears hopeless. Even the conjecture of Littré, who deletes the first μήτε and replaces the second with μεθῇ, is questionable because it calls for intervention in two places and because it is uncertain whether μεθιέναι in the sense supposed by Littré ("laisse aller le malade") can be used without an accusative object.

P. 88,5 ἰχὼρ: This word is used of the watery part of bodily liquids, e.g. of the serum of blood (see Plat., Tim. 83 c; Arist., De part. anim. II 4: 651 a 17), and of wound drainage (see e.g. Hipp., De mul. affect. I 64; II 145: VIII 130,22; 320,10 L.; Epid. VII 35: V 402,22 L.; De locis in hom. 12: VI 298,8 L.).

P. 88,9 ὠχρὸν ... ἔκλευκον: Determination of color from context is difficult. Healthy, living bone is not white, and dead bone is white only if bleached. Necrotic, infected bone is certainly not white; depending on the extent of necrosis and of infection and on the organisms involved, the infected area can be yellow or brown, and, after subsidence of infection, the dry, necrotic bone can become tan, grey or whitish. In this passage ἔκλευκος should probably be rendered "off-white" and the bone seen as buff or tan or yellowish, not very different from ὠχρός.

P. 88,9–10 ἐπὶ τῇ γλώσσῃ φλύκταιναι γίνονται: The reference may be to the lesions of herpetic or of aphthous stomatitis.

P. 88,10 σπασμὸς: See above, pp. 111–112, the note to p. 80,11–14.

P. 88,14: ἀπόπληκτοι may describe any or all of the continuum of disabilities from weakness or paralysis of one extremity to paralysis of both extremities on one side to unconsciousness with absence of all purposeful movements. The location of the sentence, following immediately the description of unilateral seizures, suggests that the author may have had in mind particularly those cases of brain injury that have contralateral seizures and contralateral paresis or paralysis.

P. 88,19 καπυρὸν: The meaning here is unsatisfactory. While exposed skull, stripped of periosteum, might well become dry and perhaps therefore be more readily abraded with a rasp, in the case presented, where the patient is febrile and the wound probably infected, one would expect the consistency of the skull, if changed at all in the acute phase of the illness, to be softer (as indicated elsewhere by the author, p. 90,29). Cornarius' conjecture, εὔπριστον in place of καπυρὸν, was apparently made in an effort to introduce an expression parallel to εὔξυστον; however, it does not solve the problem since, on the one hand, it is difficult to imagine how εὔπριστον in the course of the tradition could have been replaced by καπυρὸν, and, on the other hand, εὔξυστον, with which it is paired, also presupposes bone that is dry. But the fact that a questionable representation of the facts has been given is insufficient basis for rejection of καπυρὸν, which is supported by its occurrence elsewhere in medical texts, e.g. Diocl., fr. 147: p. 189,20 Wellmann; Dieuches, fr. 15: p. 236,10 Bertier.

P. 90,8–15: When the doctor has been in charge of the patient's care from the beginning, if trephination is called for, he should proceed cautiously and not immediately trephine to the dura and remove the bone button. Two reasons are given for leaving the bone in place: 1. the dura is less apt to be exposed to noxious influences, and 2. the dura is less apt to be damaged during surgery. Therefore, the surgeon is told to stop trephining when very little remains to be sawn through and just when the bone can be moved, and to allow the bone to separate on its own. This means that only a narrow bridge of inner table can remain connecting the bone button to the rest of the skull; perforation of the inner table must be complete for most of the circumference of the cut before any motion can be detected in the bone button. Also, of course, only a minimal bridge of inner table could be left if the bone button were to separate on its own, a bridge so thin that slight angulation of the button would sever it. In view of this, demi-trépanation, Littré's term for the procedure described in Epidemics V 16 (V 214,23–216,1 L.), where trephination was carried only through the outer table (μέχρι τῆς διπλόης), has, contrary to Littré's discussion (V 35; 198–199), no substantial support in De capitis vulneribus.

For the act of trephination the author uses the verbs πρίειν, διαπρίειν and ἐκπρίειν. πρίειν is used without regard to depth. διαπρίειν has the meaning "trephine through", indicating complete perforation of the bone to the dura. ἐκπρίειν means "trephine out", "trephine and remove", accounting for the repeated combination of ἐκπρίειν with ἀφαιρεῖν (pp. 84,20; 90,11–12. 22–23; 92,3).

P. 90,9 οὐ – 10 διεμύδησεν: The reference here is to the harmful consequences of moisture. Blood or serum pooled over the dura would in most cases in antiquity, under the conditions of wounding (low velocity weapons at normal temperature) and of wound treatment (minimal debridement), provide an ideal medium for bacterial growth and so lead to infection. This sentence recapitulates the thought expressed at p. 84,20–23.

P. 90,15 ἐν γὰρ τῷ διαπριωτῷ ὀστέῳ καὶ ἐπιλελειμμένῳ τῆς πρίσιος: In the preceding sentence the author states (lines 13–14), ἤδη κινῆται τὸ ὀστέον. By this he must mean, "when the disc of skull being excised can first be budged". Such a disc or bone button cannot be moved at all until a part of the inner table has been sawn through, completely penetrated. And no spontaneous separation of the disc would be apt to occur unless a fair amount of the inner table circumference were penetrated. Therefore, διαπριωτῷ ὀστέῳ refers to the part of the disc circumference that has been completely sawn through, while ἐπιλελειμμένῳ τῆς πρίσιος refers to the segment(s) of the circumference where a very thin layer of inner table has been left intact. The addition of οὐ before διαπριωτῷ, proposed by Littré in order that both elements describe a cut that lacks a little of being complete, is not necessary with the understanding of the text outlined above. The reasoning must be: in a case where trephining is stopped just short of complete section of the inner table and removal of the disc, no harm occurs because the part left intact is very thin and therefore presumably will break and allow the disc to separate, providing the benefit of elevation of a bony disc without the risk of complete trephination and removal of the disc.

P. 90,18 Πρίοντα – 19 ἐναποβάπτειν: This same advice on the use of hand drills is still given to beginning neurosurgical residents in the 20th c.

P. 90,25 Ἢν – 27 μήνιγγα: The obvious assumption here is that the patient was not doing well on the initial medical regimen; the author's recommendations may not have been followed, or, despite adherence to the recommended guidelines, complications may have arisen. While we now know that there may be many causes for clinical deterioration in cases of head injury (such as cerebral edema, subdural hematoma, etc.), the major complication recognized by the author of De capitis vulneribus was infection. Therefore, the reference to taking over the management of a case where treatment was begun by another doctor is important to the extent that, in the elapsed time, infection may have begun in the skull and prompt removal of the bone then became the only treatment option. Excision of a section of skull could remove infected tissue and allow drainage of blood and pus accumulated between the inner table and the dura.

P. 90,26 πρίονι ... χαρακτῷ: Since πρίων is used of a saw, an adjective which means only "toothed" would not add to the description. Obviously the meaning "sharp-toothed" is intended. In a wound where infection may already involve the bone special care is necessary because acutely infected bone is softer than healthy bone. If the saw teeth are not sharp the surgeon tends to compensate by applying more pressure to the saw. And in the case of infected bone this could result in serious injury, with the trephine plunging through the skull and lacerating the dura and even the brain.

P. 90,27 Θαμινὰ – 28 πρίονος: The author advises great caution whenever the surgeon plans to perforate the skull completely (cf. p. 92,4–5). This remains the technique for determining perforation of the inner table in trephining. The circular saw track (περίοδος) is too narrow for reliance on visual inspection, but a narrow probe inserted gently through the cut reveals at once either a firm plate of inner table or the yielding softness of the dura.

P. 90,29 ὑπόπυόν ... διάπυον: Here a real contrast seems to be intended in the use of the two words, with ὑπόπυον indicating the onset of suppuration and διάπυον an advanced stage. While it is possible that the author of De capitis vulneribus is warning the surgeon to be cautious not just in cases of frank suppuration but also in those where suppuration is just beginning, both (τε) in early and also (καὶ) in advanced cases, probably the meaning is, "in cases where suppuration has begun and is well advanced". From a practical standpoint, when cranial suppuration is evident on inspection it is usually well advanced.

P. 90,34; 92,6: ἀνακινεῖν with the meaning "to rock back and forth" accords well with a common practice in use of the trephine. When the inner table is being sawn the surgeon will periodically rock the trephine gently to and fro. As soon as the trephine has completely perforated the inner table the bone button can be felt to move with the trephine in these rocking movements. This manœuvre supplements examination by the probe in determining full perforation and can also be used in lifting out the bone button.

P. 92,3 Καὶ – 4 μήνιγγος: In this case, no reason is given for the surgeon's desire to remove skull down to dura at once. However, this decision may imply that the patient's condition is poor enough to warrant the more dangerous procedure. In this instance there would not be time enough for infection to develop. Therefore the patient's neurologic status would be the determining factor. Either his state of consciousness had deteriorated or he had developed paralysis, paresis or seizures.

P. 92,6 τρυπάνῳ: The brief mention of the perforator here probably reflects popular practice. Some surgeons undoubtedly found the perforator easier and safer to use than the trephine (see above, p. 116, the note to p. 86,30). Therefore the author of De capitis vulneribus, although preferring the trephine himself, acknowledges this practice but advises that the same care be taken in the use of the perforator as in the use of the trephine.

INDEX VERBORVM

* = exempla; → = vide

FSC
www.fsc.org
MIX
Papier | Fördert
gute Waldnutzung
FSC® C083411

Kolibri 360 GmbH
Ferdinand-Jühlke-Straße 7
99095 Erfurt, Deutschland
produktsicherheit@kolibri360.de